HOME CARE PLANNING BASED ON DRGs:
FUNCTIONAL HEALTH PATTERN MODEL

Jacqueline J. Birmingham, RN, BSN, MS
Director of Home Care
Hartford Hospital
Hartford, Connecticut

Co-published by

Fleschner Publishing Company
Bethany, CT

J. B. Lippincott Company Philadelphia
London   Mexico City   New York   St. Louis   São Paulo   Sydney

6   5   4   3   2   1

Library of Congress Cataloging in Publication Data

Birmingham, Jacqueline Joseph.
    Home care planning based on DRGs.

    Bibliography: p.
    1. Home nursing—Planning.   2. Diagnosis related
groups.   I. Title.
RT61.B57   1986   362.1'4'068   85-13092
ISBN 0-397-54563-0

The author and publisher have exerted every effort to ensure that drug selection and dosage set forth in this text are in accord with current recommendations and practice at the time of publication. However, in view of ongoing research, changes in government regulations, and the constant flow of information relating to drug therapy and drug reactions, the reader is urged to check the package insert for each drug for any change in indications and dosage and for added warnings and precautions. This is particularly important when the recommended agent is a new or infrequently employed drug.

CONTRIBUTORS

These persons contributed the chapters indicated:

MDC 04
Diseases and Disorders of the Respiratory System
Kathy Yavinsky, RN, BSN
Instructor, Staff Development
Hartford Hospital

MDC 05
Diseases and Disorders of the Circulatory System
Nancy Houle, RN, BSN
Head Nurse
Surgical Cardiology
Hartford Hospital

MDC 11
Diseases and Disorders of the Kidney and Urinary Tract
Ann Richards, RN, C, BSN
Nutritional Support Clinician
Home Care Department
Hartford Hospital

ACKNOWLEDGMENTS

These persons contributed portions of the chapters indicated:

MDC 01
Diseases and Disorders of the Nervous System
Linda Pfisterer, RN
Home Care Coordinator
Hartford Hospital

MDC 03
Diseases and Disorders of the Ear, Nose and Throat
Carole Coulom, RN, BSN, MSN
Vice President — Nursing
Visiting Nurse and Home Care, Inc.
Hartford, CT

MDC 08
Diseases and Disorders of the Musculoskeletal System and Connective Tissue
Geraldine K. Carini, RN
Orthopedic Nurse Clinician
Hartford Hospital

MDC 10
Endocrine, Nutritional and Metabolic Diseases and Disorders
Anita Gorman, RN, BSN, MS
Diabetes Clinician
Leigh Berrian, RN, BSN
Staff Nurse — Diabetes Program
Hartford Hospital

This book is dedicated to my partner at home, Ron.

TABLE OF CONTENTS

PREFACE

DRGs establish the link between diagnoses and the resources those diagnoses should consume. The *plan* for home care establishes the link between acute hospital care and home care. In the home environment, care is given intermittently as compared to a hospital where a patient is under the constant supervision of a nurse.

In a hospital setting the physician sees the patient frequently and writes orders frequently. In a home care setting it is the home health nurse who sees the patient on a regular basis and assesses the patient's progress toward established goals. Although the order for home care is the order of the physician, the plan for meeting those goals is frequently the plan of the nurse. Regardless of who is responsible for the plan of care, there must be a goal-oriented plan.

Linking DRGs with long-term planning is not a new concept. The two Yale University professors primarily responsible for the development of DRGs see in them a method of improving hospital management and precisely identifying current and long-range public health needs.

This book is designed as a resource for health professionals who need to plan home care for patients in the new arena of health care financing. It is designed to integrate the concept of organizing health care planning into categories and to determine a common need of patients based on similar diagnoses. It is designed to help care planners be cost effective.

In order to use a book which is based on DRGs, an understanding of the DRG is essential. DRG is an abbreviation for Diagnosis Related Groups. The DRG system is a classification scheme that groups short-term, general hospital patients into a manageable number of anatomically and age-related categories. The DRG system, in its present form, is primarily oriented to short-term general hospital patient populations. The DRG system is not applicable to children's hospitals, psychiatric hospitals, chronic hospitals or out-patient care. This will change! DRGs reflect medical practice in that they are organized similarly to physician specialties which are organized by anatomical organ systems.

Variables used to determine DRG classification include the principal diagnosis, other diagnoses, procedures, age and discharge status of the patient.

The system of assigning a DRG involves the patient's medical record and a computer program called **The Grouper.** There is a very intricate "decision tree" process used in The Grouper program. Since the actual DRG code is not known while the patient is still in the hospital, it is even more critical to be aware of the resources that are being consumed. It is also vital to hospitals that the diagnosis with which the patient is admitted be as accurate, concise and valid as possible.

In most cases the admitting diagnosis can be used to predict the DRG. Knowing the length of stay (LOS) allowed per DRG can help determine when the patient might be expected to be discharged. This in turn will help determine when to implement the plan.

Knowing that the hospital will be reimbursed only so much money, and that the hospital stay will only be reimbursed for so many days for each DRG is the built-in incentive for cost containment.

One feature of DRGs is **clinical coherence.** This means that when a DRG category is described to a physician, the physician will be able to identify a specific course of treatment. This same course of action must also be implemented by the nursing profession. We must be able to predict and plan home care needs.

The grouping of individual patients into one DRG is valid. It was found that individual patients in the same DRG, even though the diagnosis is somewhat different, can be expected to use a similar amount of resources.

How does the system work? Very simply stated, the system works by dividing patient admissions into Major Diagnostic Categories (MDCs), then subdividing the MDCs into subdiagnoses. The subdiagnoses are then grouped into categories by determining how much each diagnosis should cost to treat. For example, historically it was found that the cost to repair a rectocele was similar to that of a hemicolectomy; thus both diagnoses were assigned to the same group (see **DRG 149**).

It was also found that if the patient with the same procedure was 70 or older, or was less than 70 and had a complication or a coexisting diagnosis, that the **cost would be expected to be greater;** thus the case was assigned to a different group (see **DRG 148**).

There are 23 Major Diagnostic Categories (MDCs) and 467 Diagnostic Related Groups (DRGs). The number of **Medical** diagnoses and/or **Surgical** procedures varies in each DRG. The International Classification of Disease, 9th Revision: Clinical Modification (ICD-9-CM) coding scheme contains over 14,000 different diagnostic codes and over 4,000 procedure codes.

In the following work, the 23 MDCs are treated separately. The DRGs within those categories have been listed, explained and analyzed to make using this system as easy as possible.

The scope of this book is limited to the planning phase of the nursing process. The book is limited to the practice of nursing. Home care is not limited to the practice of nursing, but traditionally nurses play a vital role in coordinating, assessing and monitoring care of the patient in the home.

This book is also limited to the care of the adult patient in a medical/surgical setting. Although all DRGs are listed and described, those including pediatrics, obstetrics and mental health diagnoses are not addressed. These areas are considered specialty areas and, at the time of writing of this book, patients' hospital costs were not being paid for in a prospective payment system.

The home care needs are very different for patients in these specialties; therefore, the author recommends that readers who need more than DRG information in these categories are encouraged to consult other current references for additional information.

This book is **disease/diagnosis** oriented. It addresses the care of patients on a continuum from the acute care hospital to the home. The **plan** is focused on restorative care. Maintenance of health status is addressed only within the scope of preventing readmission to the hospital.

Nursing must become cost conscious and be able to plan for essential care. DRGs and all the issues surrounding them are not pleasant. We cannot provide everything we think would be nice for the patient. We must provide what the patient **needs** and only that! And only for as long as it is needed!

The public is demanding cost containment. If we plan carefully we can give the public what it wants without individual patient sacrifice.

INTRODUCTION

As we enter the end of the '80s, the emergence of the importance of nurses in the continuum of care is becoming more clear. In the era of cost containment the utilization of nursing services has always been and always will be a bargain.

The view of nurses as the primary health professionals in the nonacute setting has a long tradition. The agencies that have long been going into the home to provide care have been called visiting **nurse** associations. Likewise, health settings where patients receive extended care for an illness are called **nursing** homes. Nurses who give care in the home have been called various names such as Community Health Nurse, Public Health Nurse, and Home Health Nurse. The health professional with the responsibility for assessing needs of patients, planning for care, facilitating the implementation of the care and evaluation of the outcome has been the independent function of the nurse. In no other health setting does so much responsibility rest on the nurse. Indeed the physician directs the medical care and prescribes the medical therapy but the patient's health care environment is directed by a nurse.

As hospital nurses, the function of discharge planning is a part of the professional responsibility of all nurses. As the patient progresses in the hospital to a safe level of functioning to the point where he/she can go home, the hospital nurse must evaluate the total patient to help decide on the option of home care, on what the patient, family and significant others need in the home care setting.

This decision can be made in a systematic way. By using the information in this book, the patient's needs can be evaluated, related to their diagnosis and an initial plan can be made.

Why were **functional health patterns** used as a basis for this book? The underlying question for home care is not "what is the diagnosis?," but "what is the effect of the diagnosis on the patient's ability to function?"

The **functional status** or the ability to perform a specified action or activity or to carry out normal activity is the most important concern for health professionals in the home care setting. All health professionals and paraprofessionals need to know the patient's functional status when the patient is in the home care setting.

In those instances in a hospital setting where social workers do discharge planning, this book will become invaluable to them. It will give them a guide to use in conferring with the patient's primary nurse not only for planning the discharge to home but in deciding what facts need to be communicated to the person responsible for care in the home.

The functional health patterns addressed in this book have been adapted in part from work on the functional health pattern used to make nursing diagnoses (Gordon, Marjory. Nursing Diagnosis: Process and Application. McGraw-Hill. New York. 1982).

Below are listed the functional health patterns with examples of areas to be concerned with when planning for home care:

1. Health Management Deficit — will the patient's hospitalization experience change the patient's ability to carry on his/her health management from prehospital level? What effect does the hospital experience have on the patient's ability or desire to comply with his/her health care regime? Will the current hospitalization increase or decrease the potential for infection or other complications of illness?

2. Nutritional-Metabolic Pattern — will the hospital experience or discharge diagnosis change the patient's metabolic status and put him/her at risk for impaired skin integrity? Does the patient's diagnosis include a need for a change in nutritional patterns?

3. Elimination Pattern — Has there been a change in bowel and bladder function, thus a change in management of these patterns?

4. Activity and Exercise Pattern — Can the patient carry out activities of daily living whether independently, with the help of devices and/or supervision, or with physical assistance; or is the patient unable to participate at all while needing full care?

Activities which need evaluation for any patient being discharged to home include: dressing, bathing, ambulating, eating, toileting; homemaking including shopping, cooking and cleaning; and compliance with medical regime including taking prescribed medication, exercise requirements and getting medical follow-up.

5. Sleep-Rest Pattern — what are the home arrangements for sleeping? Is the bedroom easily accessible to the bathroom and kitchen facilities? Does the patient need a hospital bed and/or safety equipment? What changes in the home environment need to be made to allow for comfort for the patient?

6. Cognitive-Perceptual Pattern — does the patient, caregiver, family and/or significant others understand the disease process and the full impact of the decision for home care? Does the patient have a sensory deficit that will interfere with his/her ability to function? Is pain a factor that must be dealt with? Is the patient confused or disoriented to the point where he/she cannot function safely in the home environment?

7. Self-Perception/Self-Concept Pattern — is the patient expressing fear of the outcome of therapy or of the unknown outcome of home care arrangements? Is the patient fearful that the arrangements will be inadequate or too costly? Does the patient have altered body image or low self-esteem because of diagnosis and prognosis or as a result of visible body changes?

8. Role-Relationship Pattern — is the patient experiencing grief to the point of dysfunction? If the patient has a terminal illness, is the death and dying process in the grieving stage? Does the patient have adequate support system to handle the grieving process? Will the role relationship of parenting, spousal arrangements or role patterns with significant others be changed, or perceived to be changed because of the effect of the illness on the patient's ability to function? Is verbal communication impaired? Is there a potential for strain on the interpersonal relationships that will lead to inattentive, noncompliant, neglectful or abusive behavior by the caregiver to the patient or by the patient to the caregiver or other family members, especially adolescent children?

9. Sexuality-Reproductive Pattern — will there be an interruption in the patient/spouse/significant other sexual pattern because of the diagnosis, prognosis or ability to function? Will the patient's need for special sleeping arrangements force changes in sleeping habits? Can the patient sleep with his/her usual bed partner even though sexual intercourse is not possible? Does the reversal in caring roles impact on the patient or caregiver's feelings of sexual need or desirability? Will the patient and significant other need counseling regarding long-term changes in sexual behavior because of a permanent interruption in sexual ability?

10. Coping-Stress Tolerance Pattern — will the patient and significant others be able to cope with an illness that extends beyond the hospital stay? Did the patient anticipate the need for home care? What is the impact of a major illness on the family? Will there be significant financial requirements that will affect the family's usual lifestyle? Is this present interruption in the patient's ability to function going to affect the nuclear or extended family's ability to function?

11. Value-Belief Pattern — are the patient's or family's spiritual needs being met? Does the loss of hope affect the patient's ability to function? Will the patient and family be able to receive pastoral counseling?

In addition to assessing the functional level of the patient, the functional level of the primary caregiver must also be evaluated. All of the areas listed above must be assessed in the caregiver. It is not unusual to find the caregiver to be an elderly, frail individual with as many needs as the patient.

An assessment of availability of home care services is necessary since in a rural setting some home care services may not be readily available.

The reimbursement issue must be addressed. It is important to remember that the cost issue is why DRGs were implemented.

The cost effectiveness of home care is being evaluated. The return to a high level of family participation, or outpatient services, and the control of reimbursement for specific services and medical items are areas that will have an impact on home care.

When the nurse is planning for home care, **all** of the issues need to be addressed.

HOW TO USE THIS BOOK

Each MDC will be treated separately. Within each MDC are various numbers of DRGs. In all but two of the MDCs the DRG is classified as either **medical** or **surgical.** For example, in MDC 6, Diseases and Disorders of the Digestive System, there are 26 **surgical** and 19 **medical** DRGs.

In each chapter you will find the following information:

1. Definition of the MDC.

2. Each DRG within that MDC will be listed with a number, relative weight for dollar value (RW$), the classification (either **surgical** or **medical**), the mean length of stay (Mean LOS), outlier cutoff and name of the DRG.

The following is an example:

DRG 153

| MDC 06 | RW$ 1.2599 | Surgical | Outlier Cutoff 29 | Mean LOS 9.3 |

Minor Small and Large Bowel Procedures – Age < 70 w/o CC

In this DRG the patient has a stoma closure, is under 70 years of age and has no comorbidity or complication. He/she will have a surgical procedure and will be expected to be hospitalized approximately 9.3 days.

The hospital will be paid 1.2599 times the hospital cost-per-case rate. This cost-per-case rate is determined individually for each hospital and is calculated based on its type, region, medical education costs and other factors.

If the patient stays 29 days, which is about 20 days longer than the mean, medical review will be done to determine if the additional cost can be paid.

3. For each DRG the author has selected from the complete listing of diagnoses in that group some diagnoses that have potential home care needs. The diagnoses listed are not the total listing for each DRG but is a representative list selected from the ICD-9-CM listing (Diagnosis Related Group Health System International, Richard Averill, Project Director).

4. For each of these selected diagnoses or procedures the potential problem and plan has been discussed in relation to the patient's home care and long-term needs.

To use this book as a planning guide, first determine the Major Diagnostic Category (MDC) of your patient's diagnosis. Then determine if it is a **surgical** or **medical** classification. Refer to Table 3 to locate the DRG that contains your patient's diagnosis.

Once you have determined the probable DRG, refer to the text pages that discuss that DRG. Always start with the Master Care Planning Guide found at the beginning of each MDC. That guide contains information for all the DRGs in that category. The information following each DRG is specific to that DRG. In a few cases the patient will have multiple diagnoses, and you will need to refer to more than one DRG.

Note: you will need to become familiar with the terms in the Glossary to be able to use this book.

GLOSSARY I — TERMS RELATED TO DRGs

Clinical Coherence   a term describing a feature of the prospective payment system which utilizes DRGs. This means that if a diagnosis is described to one physician the course of therapy he or she chooses is almost the same as what another physician would choose. The plan of treatment, the cost of treatment, and the length of stay should be consistent from one physician to another.

Comorbidity   a preexisting condition that will cause an increase in hospital length of stay by at least one day in 75% of the cases. This condition exists along with the principal diagnosis.

Complication   a condition that arises during the hospital stay that prolongs hospitalization by at least one day in 75% of the cases.

CC   abbreviation meaning **comorbidity and complication.** When assigning a DRG, both comorbidity (prehospital illness) and complication (during hospital stay) have the same effect.

Decision Tree   a branching diagram designed to help a decision-maker visualize the alternatives, critical factors, risks, and information needed to formulate decisions.

Diagnosis Related Groups (DRGs)   a classification method that assigns general acute hospital inpatients into groups. Each inpatient diagnosis can be compared with others in the related group so that resource consumption can be predicted.

Grouper   a computer program designed to form a **decision tree** for grouping of related diagnoses.

ICD-9-CM   International Classification of Diseases, 9th Edition, Clinical Modification is the diagnostic classification of disease in use in the United States.

Inlier Span   the period of time covered by a single DRG-based payment (the expected length of stay). The Federal Government used a statistical formula to determine the range of days in which it is most likely that patients whose diagnosis is in that **Diagnosis Related Group** would get well enough to go to another level of care.

Length of Stay (LOS)   the phrase used when discussing how long a patient with a particular diagnosis stays in a care setting. Each **DRG** has an assigned **LOS.**

Major Diagnostic Categories (MDCs)   one of the 23 categories into which the DRGs are further divided. These are based on medical specialties. The anatomical organ systems are the bases for determining the Major Diagnostic Categories.

NEC   means "not elsewhere classified."

NOS   means "not otherwise specified." The diagnoses cannot be further defined with the information available.

Outlier   the term used when a particular case uses more than the assigned resources. A **Day Outlier** is a particular hospital admission in which the patient stayed in the hospital longer than predicted. A **Cost Outlier** is a case in which the cost for the hospital stay was greater than predicted.

Outlier Cutoff   the maximum number of days in relation to **LOS** for which hospital costs can be billed. The cost of days from the **mean length of stay** to the **cut-off day** can be negotiated, depending on the relative illness of the patient. Costs will not be paid beyond the outlier cutoff.

Primary Diagnosis   the illness that causes the patient to be most ill. The term **primary** is used when the diagnosis using the most resources is the principal admitting diagnosis.

Principal Diagnosis   the major cause of admission to the hospital.

Readmission Rate   the value determined by studying the occurrence of readmission of a patient to an acute care setting for the same diagnosis within 7 days of discharge.

Relative Weight (RW$)   using cost data from specific hospitals, depending on their category of acute or chronic, teaching or nonteaching, urban or rural, a dollar value is determined for a general hospital stay. If your hospital's dollar value is **$2,000** and your patient is admitted with **DRG 290, Thyroid Disorders,** the **LOS** is **6.0** days and dollar amount is **0.8549 × $2,000.** or **$1,709.80.** If your patient is admitted with **DRG 302, Kidney Transplant** the **LOS** is **24.1 days** and the dollar amount is **6.6322 × $2,000** or **$13,264.40.**

If the patient does not exceed the number of days allowed, but exceeds the dollar amount allowed, the case is considered a **cost outlier.** The hospital must have a review to determine if additional payment is justified.

If the patient leaves and the stay does not cost **$1,709.80** or **$13,264.40,** the hospital is still paid that amount of money.

Resource Consumption   total cost of hospital care per admission including length of stay and other charges such as operating room, laboratory tests, drugs and solutions. Each DRG has a cost value which predicts the cost of each hospitalization. DRG cost analysis takes into account regional differences and educational needs. Because of this variation, cost information is not included in this book. It is suggested that individual health care institutions provide this basic cost information to increase awareness of and attention to the need for cost consciousness and containment.

W/O   means "without."

<70   symbol meaning less than 70 years in age. Note the symbol resembles an upper case L for less than.

>=70   symbol meaning more than or equal to 70 years of age.

>=70 and/or CC   symbol phrase meaning the DRG pertains to a patient who is **70 or older,** with or without a complication or comorbidity, or to a patient **under 70 with a complication or comorbidity.**

GLOSSARY II — TERMS RELATED TO HOME CARE

Discharge Planning the process by which plans are made by an agency to facilitate a safe, timely and cost effective discharge of a patient to either a home care setting or an extended care facility.

Durable Medical Equipment (DME) a piece of equipment that can be rented or purchased that will last the duration of an illness, in contrast to medical/surgical supplies which are disposable. It is primarily and customarily used to serve a medical purpose. It is not useful to a person in the absence of an illness or injury and it can be used in the home.

Extended Care Facility a service-oriented institution which provides health care less extensively than an acute care hospital (i.e. nursing home, hospice hospital, etc.).

Home Care the method of health care delivery in which the services are rendered for an essentially home-bound patient.

Primary Caregiver person who will be responsible for care of the patient on a 24-hour basis at home. A spouse, child, sibling or other responsible person (RP). Not all home care patients will have a Primary Caregiver.

Primary Home Care Nurse a professional nurse who is associated with a community agency, either public or private, who is responsible for assessing, planning, implementing and evaluating the care of the patient in his/her home environment.

Responsible Person (RP) a person who is legally responsible for the care of another person.

Significant Other (SO) a person who may or may not be legally responsible for the care of another, but who has a significant relationship with the person and can usually be included in the person's care. The SO has a choice about involvement in care.

Skilled Services services rendered by a health care professional. This includes, for example: nursing, physical therapy, medical social worker, occupational and speech therapy. Other services given in the home are homemaker and home health aides who are paraprofessionals usually working under the direction of a nurse.

TABLE 1

MDC #	Major Diagnostic Categories (MDCs)	No. of DRGs		
		Surgical	Medical	Total
1	Diseases and Disorders of the Nervous System	8	27	35
2	Diseases and Disorders of the Eye	7	6	13
3	Diseases and Disorders of the Ear, Nose and Throat	15	11	26
4	Diseases and Disorders of the Respiratory System	3	25	28
5	Diseases and Disorders of the Circulatory System	18	25	43
6	Diseases and Disorders of the Digestive System	26	19	45
7	Diseases and Disorders of the Hepatobiliary System and Pancreas	11	7	18
8	Diseases and Disorders of the Musculoskeletal System and Connective Tissue	26	22	48
9	Diseases and Disorders of the Skin, Subcutaneous Tissue and Breast	14	14	28
10	Endocrine, Nutritional and Metabolic Diseases and Disorders	9	8	17
11	Diseases and Disorders of the Kidney and Urinary Tract	14	18	32
12	Diseases and Disorders of the Male Reproductive System	12	7	19
13	Diseases and Disorders of the Female Reproductive System	13	4	17
14	Pregnancy, Childbirth and Puerperium	5	10	15
15	Newborns and Other Neonates with Conditions Originating in the Perinatal Period	NOS	NOS	7
16	Diseases and Disorders of the Blood and Blood-Forming Organs and Immunity Disorders	3	5	8
17	Myeloproliferative Disease and Disorders, Poorly Differentiated Malignancy and Other Neoplasms NEC	6	9	15
18	Infectious and Parasitic Diseases (Systemic or Unspecified Sites)	1	8	9
19	Mental Diseases and Disorders	1	8	9
20	Substance Use and Substance-Induced Organic Mental Disorders	NOS	NOS	6
21	Injury, Poisoning and Toxic Effects of Drugs	5	12	17
22	Burns	2	3	5
23	Factors Influencing Health Status and Other Contacts with Health Service	1	6	7
	SUBTOTAL for Specific DRGs			467
	There are 3 DRGs which are used for cases in which another specific DRG cannot be assigned.			3
	TOTAL			470

TABLE 2

Listing of 467 Diagnosis Related Groups

MDC 01   DISEASES AND DISORDERS OF THE NERVOUS SYSTEM

S-001	Craniotomy – Age > = 18 Except for Trauma
S-002	Craniotomy for Trauma – Age > = 18
S-003	Craniotomy – Age < 18
S-004	Spinal Procedures
S-005	Extracranial Vascular Procedures
S-006	Carpal Tunnel Release
S-007	Peripheral and Cranial Nerve & Other Nervous System Procedures Age > = 70 and/or CC
S-008	Peripheral and Cranial Nerve & Other Nervous System Procedures – Age < 70 w/o CC
M-009	Spinal Disorders and Injuries
M-010	Nervous System Neoplasms – Age > = 70 and/or CC
M-011	Nervous System Neoplasms – Age < 70 w/o CC
M-012	Degenerative Nervous System Disorders
M-013	Multiple Sclerosis and Cerebellar Ataxia
M-014	Specific Cerebrovascular Disorders Except Transient Ischemic Attacks
M-015	Transient Ischemic Attacks
M-016	Nonspecific Cerebrovascular Disorders with CC
M-017	Nonspecific Cerebrovascular Disorders w/o CC
M-018	Cranial and Peripheral Nerve Disorders – Age > = 70 and/or CC
M-019	Cranial and Peripheral Nerve Disorders – Age < 70 w/o CC
M-020	Nervous System Infection Except Viral Meningitis
M-021	Viral Meningitis
M-022	Hypertensive Encephalopathy
M-023	Nontraumatic Stupor and Coma
M-024	Seizure and Headache – Age > = 70 and/or CC
M-025	Seizure and Headache – Age 18–69 w/o CC
M-026	Seizure and Headache – Age 0–17
M-027	Traumatic Stupor and Coma, Coma > 1 hour
M-028	Traumatic Stupor and Coma, Coma < 1 hour – Age > = 70 and/or CC
M-029	Traumatic Stupor and Coma < 1 hour – Age 18–69 w/o CC
M-030	Traumatic Stupor and Coma < 1 hour – Age 0–17
M-031	Concussion – Age > = 70 and/or CC
M-032	Concussion – Age 18–69 w/o CC
M-033	Concussion – Age 0–17
M-034	Other Disorders of the Nervous System – Age > = 70 and/or CC
M-035	Other Disorders of the Nervous System – Age < 70 w/o CC

MDC 02   DISEASES AND DISORDERS OF THE EYE

S-036   Retinal Procedures

S-037   Orbital Procedures

S-038   Primary Iris Procedures

S-039   Lens Procedures

S-040   Extraocular Procedures Except Orbit – Age > = 18

S-041   Extraocular Procedures Except Orbit – Age 0–17

S-042   Intraocular Procedures Except Retina, Iris and Lens

M-043   Hyphema

M-044   Acute Major Eye Infections

M-045   Neurological Eye Disorders

M-046   Other Disorders of the Eye – Age > = 18 with CC

M-047   Other Disorders of the Eye – Age > = 18 w/o CC

M-048   Other Disorders of the Eye – Age 0–17

MDC 03   DISEASES AND DISORDERS OF THE EAR, NOSE AND THROAT

S-049   Major Head and Neck Procedures

S-050   Sialoadenectomy

S-051   Salivary Gland Procedures Except Sialoadenectomy

S-052   Cleft Lip and Palate Repair

S-053   Sinus and Mastoid Procedures – Age > = 18

S-054   Sinus and Mastoid Procedures – Age 0–17

S-055   Miscellaneous Ear, Nose and Throat Procedures

S-056   Rhinoplasty

S-057   Tonsillectomy and Adenoidectomy Procedure Except Tonsillectomy and/or Adenoidectomy – Age > = 18

S-058   Tonsillectomy and Adenoidectomy Procedure Except Tonsillectomy and/or Adenoidectomy – Age 0–17

S-059   Tonsillectomy and/or Adenoidectomy – Age > = 18

S-060   Tonsillectomy and/or Adenoidectomy – Age 0–17

S-061   Myringotomy – Age > = 18

S-062   Myringotomy – Age 0–17

S-063   Other Ear, Nose and Throat Operating Room Procedures

M-064   Ear, Nose and Throat Malignancy

M-065   Dysequilibrium

M-066   Epistaxis

M-067   Epiglottitis

M-068   Otitis Media and Upper Respiratory Infection – Age > = 70 and/or CC

M-069   Otitis Media and Upper Respiratory Infection – Age 18–69 w/o CC

M-070   Otitis Media and Upper Respiratory Infection – Age 0–17

M-071   Laryngotracheitis

M-072   Nasal Trauma and Deformity

M-073   Other Ear, Nose and Throat Diagnoses – Age > = 18

M-074   Other Ear, Nose and Throat Diagnoses – Age 0–17

MDC 04 DISEASES AND DISORDERS OF THE RESPIRATORY SYSTEM

S-075   Major Chest Procedures
S-076   Operating Room Procedures on the Respiratory System Except Major Chest with CC
S-077   Operating Room Procedures on the Respiratory System Except Major Chest w/o CC
M-078   Pulmonary Embolism
M-079   Respiratory Infections and Inflammations – Age > = 70 and/or CC
M-080   Respiratory Infections and Inflammations – Age 18–69 w/o CC
M-081   Respiratory Infections and Inflammations – Age 0–17
M-082   Respiratory Neoplasms
M-083   Major Chest Trauma – Age > = 70 and/or CC
M-084   Major Chest Trauma – Age < 70 w/o CC
M-085   Pleural Effusion – Age > = 70 and/or CC
M-086   Pleural Effusion – Age < 70 w/o CC
M-087   Pulmonary Edema and Respiratory Failure
M-088   Chronic Obstructive Pulmonary Disease
M-089   Simple Pneumonia and Pleurisy – Age > = 70 and/or CC
M-090   Simple Pneumonia and Pleurisy – Age 18–69 w/o CC
M-091   Simple Pneumonia and Pleurisy – Age 0–17
M-092   Interstitial Lung Disease – Age > = 70 and/or CC
M-093   Interstitial Lung Disease – Age < 70 w/o CC
M-094   Pneumothorax – Age > = 70 and/or CC
M-095   Pneumothorax – Age < 70 w/o CC
M-096   Bronchitis and Asthma – Age > = 70 and/or CC
M-097   Bronchitis and Asthma – Age 18–69 w/o CC
M-098   Bronchitis and Asthma – Age 0–17
M-099   Respiratory Signs and Symptoms – Age > = 70 and/or CC
M-100   Respiratory Signs and Symptoms – Age < 70 w/o CC
M-101   Other Respiratory Diagnoses – Age > = 70 and/or CC
M-102   Other Respiratory Diagnoses – Age < 70

MDC 05 DISEASES AND DISORDERS OF THE CIRCULATORY SYSTEM

S-103   Heart Transplant
S-104   Cardiac Valve Procedure with Pump and with Cardiac Catheterization
S-105   Cardiac Valve Procedure with Pump and w/o Cardiac Catheterization
S-106   Coronary Bypass with Cardiac Catheterization
S-107   Coronary Bypass w/o Cardiac Catheterization
S-108   Cardiothoracic Procedures, Except Valve and Coronary Bypass, with Pump
S-109   Cardiothoracic Procedures w/o Pump
S-110   Major Reconstructive Vascular Procedures – Age > = 70 and/or CC
S-111   Major Reconstructive Vascular Procedures – Age < 70 w/o CC
S-112   Vascular Procedures Except Major Reconstruction
S-113   Amputation for Circulatory System Disorders Except Upper Limb and Toe
S-114   Upper Limb and Toe Amputation for Circulatory System Disorders
S-115   Permanent Cardiac Pacemaker Implant with AMI or CHF

S-116	Permanent Cardiac Pacemaker Implant w/o AMI or CHF
S-117	Cardiac Pacemaker Replacement and Revision Excluding Pulse Generator Replacement Only
S-118	Cardiac Pacemaker Pulse Generator Replacement Only
S-119	Vein Ligation and Stripping
S-120	Other Operating Room Procedures on the Circulatory System
M-121	Circulatory Disorders with AMI and Cardiovascular Complications, Discharged Alive
M-122	Circulatory Disorders with AMI w/o Cardiovascular Complications, Discharged Alive
M-123	Circulatory Disorders with AMI, Expired
M-124	Circulatory Disorders Excluding AMI, with Cardiac Catheterization and Complex Diagnosis
M-125	Circulatory Disorders Excluding AMI, with Cardiac Catheterization w/o Complex Diagnosis
M-126	Acute and Subacute Endocarditis
M-127	Heart Failure and Shock
M-128	Deep Vein Thrombophlebitis
M-129	Cardiac Arrest
M-130	Peripheral Vascular Disorders – Age > = 70 and/or CC
M-131	Peripheral Vascular Disorders – Age < 70 w/o CC
M-132	Atherosclerosis – Age > = 70 and/or CC
M-133	Atherosclerosis – Age < 70 w/o CC
M-134	Hypertension
M-135	Cardiac Congenital and Valvular Disorders – Age > = 70 and/or CC
M-136	Cardiac Congenital and Valvular Disorders – Age 18–69 w/o CC
M-137	Cardiac Congenital and Valvular Disorders – Age 0–17
M-138	Cardiac Arrhythmia and Conduction Disorders – Age > = 70 and/or CC
M-139	Cardiac Arrhythmia and Conduction Disorders – Age < 70 w/o CC
M-140	Angina Pectoris
M-141	Syncope and Collapse – Age > = 70 and/or CC
M-142	Syncope and Collapse – Age < 70 w/o CC
M-143	Chest Pain
M-144	Other Circulatory Diagnoses with CC
M-145	Other Circulatory Diagnoses w/o CC

MDC 06 DISEASES AND DISORDERS OF THE DIGESTIVE SYSTEM

S-146	Rectal Resection – Age > = 70 and/or CC
S-147	Rectal Resection – Age < 70 w/o CC
S-148	Major Small and Large Bowel Procedures – Age > = 70 and/or CC
S-149	Major Small and Large Bowel Procedures – Age < 70 w/o CC
S-150	Peritoneal Adhesiolysis – Age > = 70 and/or CC
S-151	Peritoneal Adhesiolysis – Age < 70 w/o CC
S-152	Minor Small and Large Bowel Procedures – Age > = 70 and/or CC
S-153	Minor Small and Large Bowel Procedures – Age < 70 w/o CC
S-154	Stomach, Esophageal and Duodenal Procedures – Age > = 70 and/or CC
S-155	Stomach, Esophageal and Duodenal Procedures – Age 18–69 w/o CC

S-156	Stomach, Esophageal and Duodenal Procedures – Age 0–17
S-157	Anal Procedures – Age $\geq$ 70 and/or CC
S-158	Anal Procedures – Age < 70 w/o CC
S-159	Hernia Procedures Except Inguinal and Femoral – Age $\geq$ 70 and/or CC
S-160	Hernia Procedures Except Inguinal and Femoral – Age 18–69 w/o CC
S-161	Inguinal and Femoral Hernia Procedures – Age $\geq$ 70 and/or CC
S-162	Inguinal and Femoral Hernia Procedures – Age 18–69 w/o CC
S-163	Hernia Procedures – Age 0–17
S-164	Appendectomy with Complicated Principal Diagnosis – Age $\geq$ 70 and/or CC
S-165	Appendectomy with Complicated Principal Diagnosis – Age < 70 w/o CC
S-166	Appendectomy w/o Complicated Principal Diagnosis – Age $\geq$ 70 and/or CC
S-167	Appendectomy w/o Complicated Principal Diagnosis – Age < 70 w/o CC
S-168	Procedures on the Mouth – Age $\geq$ 70 and/or CC
S-169	Procedures on the Mouth – Age < 70 w/o CC
S-170	Other Digestive System Procedures – Age $\geq$ 70 and/or CC
S-171	Other Digestive System Procedures – Age < 70 w/o CC
M-172	Digestive Malignancy – Age $\geq$ 70 and/or CC
M-173	Digestive Malignancy – Age < 70 w/o CC
M-174	GI Hemorrhage – Age $\geq$ 70 and/or CC
M-175	GI Hemorrhage – Age < 70 w/o CC
M-176	Complicated Peptic Ulcer
M-177	Uncomplicated Peptic Ulcer – Age $\geq$ 70 and/or CC
M-178	Uncomplicated Peptic Ulcer – Age < 70 w/o CC
M-179	Inflammatory Bowel Disease
M-180	GI Obstruction – Age $\geq$ 70 and/or CC
M-181	GI Obstruction – Age < 70 w/o CC
M-182	Esophagitis, Gastroenteritis and Miscellaneous Digestive Disorders Age $\geq$ 70 and/or CC
M-183	Esophagitis, Gastroenteritis and Miscellaneous Digestive Disorders – Age 18–69 w/o CC
M-184	Esophagitis, Gastroenteritis and Miscellaneous Digestive Disorders – Age 0–17
M-185	Dental and Oral Disorders, Excluding Extractions and Restorations – Age $\geq$ 18
M-186	Dental and Oral Disorders, Excluding Extractions and Restorations – Age 0–17
M-187	Dental Extractions and Restorations
M-188	Other Digestive System Diagnoses – Age $\geq$ 70 and/or CC
M-189	Other Digestive System Diagnoses – Age 18–69 w/o CC
M-190	Other Digestive System Diagnoses – Age 0–17

MDC 07 DISEASES AND DISORDERS OF THE HEPATOBILIARY SYSTEM, PANCREAS

S-191	Major Pancreas, Liver and Shunt Procedures
S-192	Minor Pancreas, Liver and Shunt Procedures
S-193	Biliary Tract Procedures, Excluding Total Cholecystectomy – Age $\geq$ 70 and/or CC
S-194	Biliary Tract Procedures, Excluding Total Cholecystectomy – Age < 70 w/o CC
S-195	Total Cholecystectomy with CDE – Age $\geq$ 70 and/or CC
S-196	Total Cholecystectomy with CDE – Age < 70 w/o CC

S-197	Total Cholecystectomy w/o CDE – Age > = 70 and/or CC
S-198	Total Cholecystectomy w/o CDE – Age < 70 w/o CC
S-199	Hepatobiliary Diagnostic Procedure for Malignancy
S-200	Hepatobiliary Diagnostic Procedure for Nonmalignancy
S-201	Other Hepatobiliary or Pancreas Operating Room Procedures
M-202	Cirrhosis and Alcoholic Hepatitis
M-203	Malignancy of Hepatobiliary System or Pancreas
M-204	Disorders of Pancreas Except Malignancy
M-205	Disorders of Liver Excluding Malignancy, Cirrhosis, Alcoholic Hepatitis Age > = 70 and/or CC
M-206	Disorders of Liver Excluding Malignancy, Cirrhosis, Alcoholic Hepatitis Age < 70 w/o CC
M-207	Disorders of the Biliary Tract – Age > = 70 and/or CC
M-208	Disorders of the Biliary Tract – Age < 70 w/o CC

MDC 08 DISEASES AND DISORDERS OF THE MUSCULOSKELETAL SYSTEM AND CONNECTIVE TISSUE

S-209	Major Joint Procedures
S-210	Hip and Femur Procedures Except Major Joint – Age > = 70 and/or CC
S-211	Hip and Femur Procedures Except Major Joint – Age 18–69 w/o CC
S-212	Hip and Femur Procedures Except Major Joint – Age 0–17
S-213	Amputations for Musculoskeletal System and Connective Tissue Disorders
S-214	Back and Neck Procedures – Age > = 70 and/or CC
S-215	Back and Neck Procedures – Age < 70 w/o CC
S-216	Biopsies of Musculoskeletal System and Connective Tissue
S-217	Wound Debridement and Skin Graft, Excluding Hand, for Musculoskeletal and Connective Tissue Disorders
S-218	Lower Extremities and Humerus Procedures, Excluding Hip, Foot, and Femur Age > = 70 and/or CC
S-219	Lower Extremities and Humerus Procedures, Excluding Hip, Foot and Femur Age 18–69 w/o CC
S-220	Lower Extremities and Humerus Procedures, Excluding Hip, Foot and Femur – Age 0–17
S-221	Knee Procedures – Age > = 70 and/or CC
S-222	Knee Procedures – Age < 70 w/o CC
S-223	Upper Extremity Procedures, Excluding Humerus and Hand – Age > = 70 and/or CC
S-224	Upper Extremity Procedures, Excluding Humerus and Hand – Age < 70 w/o CC
S-225	Foot Procedures
S-226	Soft Tissue Procedures – Age > = 70 and/or CC
S-227	Soft Tissue Procedures – Age < 70 w/o CC
S-228	Ganglion (Hand) Procedures
S-229	Hand Procedures, Except Ganglion
S-230	Local Excision and Removal of Internal Fixed Devices of Hip and Femur
S-231	Local Excision and Removal of Internal Fixed Devices Except Hip and Femur
S-232	Arthroscopy

S-233	Other Musculoskeletal System and Connective Tissue Operating Room Procedures Age > = 70 and/or CC
S-234	Other Musculoskeletal System and Connective Tissue Operating Room Procedures Age < 70 w/o CC
M-235	Fractures of Femur
M-236	Fractures of Hip and Pelvis
M-237	Sprains, Strains and Dislocations of Hip, Pelvis and Thigh
M-238	Osteomyelitis
M-239	Pathological Fractures and Musculoskeletal and Connective Tissue Malignancy
M-240	Connective Tissue Disorders – Age > = 70 and/or CC
M-241	Connective Tissue Disorders – Age < 70 w/o CC
M-242	Septic Arthritis
M-243	Medical Back Problems
M-244	Bone Diseases and Septic Arthropathy – Age > = 70 and/or CC
M-245	Bone Diseases and Septic Arthropathy – Age < 70 w/o CC
M-246	Nonspecific Arthropathies
M-247	Signs and Symptoms of Musculoskeletal System and Connective Tissue
M-248	Tendonitis, Myositis and Bursitis
M-249	Aftercare, Musculoskeletal System and Connective Tissue
M-250	Fractures, Sprains, Strains and Dislocations of Forearm, Hand, Foot Age > = 70 and/or CC
M-251	Fractures, Sprains, Strains and Dislocations of Forearm, Hand, Foot – Age 18–69 w/o CC
M-252	Fractures, Sprains, Strains and Dislocations of Forearm, Hand, Foot – Age 0–17
M-253	Fractures, Sprains, Strains and Dislocations of Upper Arm, Lower Leg, Excluding Foot Age > = 70 and/or CC
M-254	Fractures, Sprains, Strains and Dislocations of Upper Arm, Lower Leg, Excluding Foot Age 18–69 w/o CC
M-255	Fractures, Sprains, Strains and Dislocations of Upper Arm, Lower Leg, Excluding Foot Age 0–17
M-256	Other Diagnoses of Musculoskeletal System and Connective Tissue

MDC 09 DISEASES AND DISORDERS OF THE SKIN, SUBCUTANEOUS TISSUE AND BREAST

S-257	Total Mastectomy for Malignancy – Age > = 70 and/or CC
S-258	Total Mastectomy for Malignancy – Age < 70 w/o CC
S-259	Subtotal Mastectomy for Malignancy – Age > = 70 and/or CC
S-260	Subtotal Mastectomy for Malignancy – Age < 70
S-261	Breast Procedure for Nonmalignancy Except Biopsy and Local Excision
S-262	Breast Biopsy and Local Excision for Nonmalignancy
S-263	Skin Grafts for Skin Ulcer or Cellulitis – Age > = 70 and/or CC
S-264	Skin Grafts for Skin Ulcer or Cellulitis – Age < 70 w/o CC
S-265	Skin Grafts Except for Skin Ulcer or Cellulitis with CC
S-266	Skin Grafts Except for Skin Ulcer or Cellulitis w/o CC
S-267	Perianal and Pilonidal Procedures
S-268	Skin, Subcutaneous Tissue and Breast Plastic Procedures

S-269	Other Skin, Subcutaneous Tissue and Breast Operating Room Procedures Age > = 70 and/or CC
S-270	Other Skin, Subcutaneous Tissue and Breast Operating Room Procedures Age < 70 w/o CC
M-271	Skin Ulcers
M-272	Major Skin Disorders – Age > = 70 and/or CC
M-273	Major Skin Disorders – Age < 70 w/o CC
M-274	Malignant Breast Disorders – Age > = 70 and/or CC
M-275	Malignant Breast Disorders – Age < 70 w/o CC
M-276	Nonmalignant Breast Disorders
M-277	Cellulitis – Age > = 70 and/or CC
M-278	Cellulitis – Age 18–69 w/o CC
M-279	Cellulitis – Age 0–17
M-280	Trauma to the Skin, Subcutaneous Tissue and Breast – Age > = 70 and/or CC
M-281	Trauma to the Skin, Subcutaneous Tissue and Breast – Age 18–69 w/o CC
M-282	Trauma to the Skin, Subcutaneous Tissue and Breast – Age 0–17
M-283	Minor Skin Disorders – Age > = 70 and/or CC
M-284	Minor Skin Disorders – Age < 70 w/o CC

MDC 10 ENDOCRINE, NUTRITIONAL AND METABOLIC DISEASES AND DISORDERS

S-285	Amputations for Endocrine, Nutritional and Metabolic Disorders
S-286	Adrenal and Pituitary Procedures
S-287	Skin Grafts and Wound Debridement for Endocrine, Nutritional and Metabolic Disorders
S-288	Operating Room Procedures for Obesity
S-289	Parathyroid Procedures
S-290	Thyroid Procedures
S-291	Thyroglossal Procedures
S-292	Other Endocrine, Nutritional and Metabolic Operating Room Procedures Age > = 70 and/or CC
S-293	Other Endocrine, Nutritional and Metabolic Operating Room Procedures Age < 70 w/o CC
M-294	Diabetes – Age > = 36
M-295	Diabetes – Age 0–35
M-296	Nutritional and Miscellaneous Metabolic Disorders – Age > = 70 and/or CC
M-297	Nutritional and Miscellaneous Metabolic Disorders – Age 18–69 w/o CC
M-298	Nutritional and Miscellaneous Metabolic Disorders – Age 0–17
M-299	Inborn Errors of Metabolism
M-300	Endocrine Disorders – Age > = 70 and/or CC
M-301	Endocrine Disorders – Age > 70 w/o CC

MDC 11 DISEASES AND DISORDERS OF THE KIDNEY AND URINARY TRACT

S-302	Kidney Transplant
S-303	Kidney, Ureter and Major Bladder Procedure for Neoplasm
S-304	Kidney, Ureter and Major Bladder Procedure for Nonmalignancy Age > = 70 and/or CC

S-305	Kidney, Ureter and Major Bladder Procedure for Nonmalignancy – Age < 70 w/o CC
S-306	Prostatectomy – Age > = 70 and/or CC
S-307	Prostatectomy – Age < 70 w/o CC
S-308	Minor Bladder Procedures – Age > = 70 and/or CC
S-309	Minor Bladder Procedures – Age < 70 w/o CC
S-310	Transurethral Procedures – Age > = 70 and/or CC
S-311	Transurethral Procedures – Age < 70 w/o CC
S-312	Urethral Procedures – Age > = 70 and/or CC
S-313	Urethral Procedures – Age 18–69 w/o CC
S-314	Urethral Procedures – Age 0–17
S-315	Other Kidney and Urinary Tract Operating Room Procedures
M-316	Renal Failure w/o Dialysis
M-317	Renal Failure with Dialysis
M-318	Kidney and Urinary Tract Neoplasms – Age > = 70 and/or CC
M-319	Kidney and Urinary Tract Neoplasms – Age < 70 w/o CC
M-320	Kidney and Urinary Tract Infections – Age > = 70 and/or CC
M-321	Kidney and Urinary Tract Infections – Age 18–69 w/o CC
M-322	Kidney and Urinary Tract Infections – Age 0–17
M-323	Urinary Stones – Age > = 70 and/or CC
M-324	Urinary Stones – Age < 70 w/o CC
M-325	Kidney and Urinary Tract Signs and Symptoms – Age > = 70 and/or CC
M-326	Kidney and Urinary Tract Signs and Symptoms – Age 18–69 w/o CC
M-327	Kidney and Urinary Tract Signs and Symptoms – Age 0–17
M-328	Urethral Stricture – Age > = 70 and/or CC
M-329	Urethral Stricture – Age 18–69 w/o CC
M-330	Urethral Stricture – Age 0–17
M-331	Other Kidney and Urinary Tract Diagnoses – Age > = 70 and/or CC
M-332	Other Kidney and Urinary Tract Diagnoses – Age 18–69 w/o CC
M-333	Other Kidney and Urinary Tract Diagnoses – Age 0–17

MDC 12   DISEASES AND DISORDERS OF THE MALE REPRODUCTIVE SYSTEM

S-334	Major Male Pelvic Procedures with CC
S-335	Major Male Pelvic Procedures w/o CC
S-336	Transurethral Prostatectomy – Age > = 70 and/or CC
S-337	Transurethral Prostatectomy – Age < 70 w/o CC
S-338	Testes Procedures, for Malignancy
S-339	Testes Procedures, Nonmalignant – Age > = 18
S-340	Testes Procedures, Nonmalignant – Age 0–17
S-341	Penis Procedures
S-342	Circumcision – Age > = 18
S-343	Circumcision – age 0–17
S-344	Other Male Reproductive System Operating Room Procedures for Malignancy
S-345	Other Male Reproductive System Operating Room Procedures Except for Malignancy
M-346	Malignancy, Male Reproductive System – Age > = 70 and/or CC

M-347	Malignancy, Male Reproductive System – Age < 70 w/o CC
M-348	Benign Prostatic Hypertrophy – Age > = 70 and/or CC
M-349	Benign Prostatic Hypertrophy – Age < 70 w/o CC
M-350	Inflammation of the Male Reproductive System
M-351	Sterilization, Male
M-352	Other Male Reproductive System Diagnoses

MDC 13 DISEASES AND DISORDERS OF THE FEMALE REPRODUCTIVE SYSTEM

S-353	Pelvic Evisceration, Radical Hysterectomy and Vulvectomy
S-354	Nonradical Hysterectomy – Age > = 70 and/or CC
S-355	Nonradical Hysterectomy – Age < 70 w/o CC
S-356	Female Reproductive System Reconstructive Procedures
S-357	Uterus and Adnexa Procedures, for Malignancy
S-358	Uterus and Adnexa Procedures for Nonmalignancy Except Tubal Interruption
S-359	Tubal Interruption for Nonmalignancy
S-360	Vagina, Cervix and Vulva Procedures
S-361	Laparoscopy and Endoscopy (female) Except Tubal Interruption
S-362	Laparoscopic Tubal Interruption
S-363	D and C Conization and Radioimplant for Malignancy
S-364	D and C Conization Except for Malignancy
S-365	Other Female Reproductive System Operating Room Procedures
M-366	Malignancy, Female Reproductive System – Age > = 70 and/or CC
M-367	Malignancy, Female Reproductive System – Age < 70 w/o CC
M-368	Infections, Female Reproductive System
M-369	Menstrual and Other Female Reproductive System Disorders

MDC 14 PREGNANCY, CHILDBIRTH AND THE PUERPERIUM

S-370	Cesarean Section with CC
S-371	Cesarean Section w/o CC
M-372	Vaginal Delivery with Complicating Diagnoses
M-373	Vaginal Delivery w/o Complicating Diagnoses
S-374	Vaginal Delivery with Sterilization and/or D & C
S-375	Vaginal Delivery with Operating Room Procedures Except Sterilization and/or D & C
M-376	Postpartum Diagnoses w/o Operating Room Procedures
S-377	Postpartum Diagnoses with Operating Room Procedures
M-378	Ectopic Pregnancy
M-379	Threatened Abortion
M-380	Abortion w/o D & C
M-381	Abortion with D & C
M-382	False Labor
M-383	Other Antepartum Diagnoses with Medical Complications
M-384	Other Antepartum Diagnoses w/o Medical Complications

MDC 15 NEWBORNS AND OTHER NEONATES WITH CONDITIONS ORIGINATING IN THE PERINATAL PERIOD: NOS*

NOS-385 Neonates, Died or Transferred

NOS-386 Extreme Immaturity, Neonate

NOS-387 Prematurity with Major Problems

NOS-388 Prematurity w/o Major Problems

NOS-389 Full-Term Neonate with Major Problems

NOS-390 Neonates with Other Significant Problems

NOS-391 Normal Newborns

(*NOS — not otherwise specified as Surgical or Medical)

MDC 16 DISEASES AND DISORDERS OF BLOOD AND BLOOD-FORMING ORGANS

S-392 Splenectomy – Age > = 18

S-393 Splenectomy – Age 0–17

S-394 Other Operating Room Procedures of the Blood and Blood-Forming Organs

M-395 Red Blood Cell Disorders – Age > = 18

M-396 Red Blood Cell Disorders – Age 0–17

M-397 Coagulation Disorders

M-398 Reticuloendothelial and Immunity Disorders – Age > = 70 and/or CC

M-399 Reticuloendothelial and Immunity Disorders – Age < 70 w/o CC

MDC 17 MYELOPROLIFERATIVE DISORDERS

S-400 Lymphoma or Leukemia with Major Operating Room Procedure

S-401 Lymphoma or Leukemia with Minor Operating Room Procedure – Age > = 70 and/or CC

S-402 Lymphoma or Leukemia with Minor Operating Room Procedure – Age < 70 w/o CC

M-403 Lymphoma or Leukemia – Age > = 70 and/or CC

M-404 Lymphoma or Leukemia – Age 18–69 w/o CC

M-405 Lymphoma or Leukemia – Age 0–17

S-406 Myeloproliferative Disorders or Poorly Differentiated Neoplasm with Major Operating Room Procedure and CC

S-407 Myeloproliferative Disorders or Poorly Differentiated Neoplasm with Major Operating Room Procedure w/o CC

S-408 Myeloproliferative Disorders or Poorly Differentiated Neoplasm with Minor Operating Room Procedure

M-409 Radiotherapy

M-410 Chemotherapy

M-411 History of Malignancy w/o Endoscopy

M-412 History of Malignancy with Endoscopy

M-413 Other Myeloproliferative Disorders or Poorly Differentiated Neoplasm Diagnosis Age > = 70 and/or CC

M-414 Other Myeloproliferative Disorders or Poorly Differentiated Neoplasm Diagnosis Age < 70 w/o CC

MDC 18 INFECTIOUS AND PARASITIC DISEASES

S-415   Operating Room Procedure for Infectious and Parasitic Diseases
M-416   Septicemia – Age $> = 18$
M-417   Septicemia – Age 0–17
M-418   Postoperative and Posttraumatic Infections
M-419   Fever of Unknown Origin – Age $> = 70$ and/or CC
M-420   Fever of Unknown Origin – Age 18–69 w/o CC
M-421   Viral Illness – Age $> = 18$
M-422   Viral Illness and Fever of Unknown Origin – Age 0–17
M-423   Other Infectious and Parasitic Diseases Diagnoses

MDC 19 MENTAL DISEASES AND DISORDERS

S-424   Operating Room Procedures with Principal Diagnoses of Mental Illness
M-425   Acute Adjustment Reactions and Disturbances of Psychosocial Dysfunction
M-426   Depressive Neuroses
M-427   Neuroses Except Depressive
M-428   Disorders of Personality and Impulse Control
M-429   Organic Disturbances and Mental Retardation
M-430   Psychoses
M-431   Childhood Mental Disorders
M-432   Other Diagnoses of Mental Disorders

MDC 20 SUBSTANCE USE AND SUBSTANCE-INDUCED ORGANIC MENTAL DISORDERS — NOS*

NOS-433 Substance Use and Substance-Induced Organic Mental Disorders, Left Against Medical Advice
NOS-434 Drug Dependence
NOS-435 Drug Use Except Dependence
NOS-436 Alcohol Dependence
NOS-437 Alcohol Use Except Dependence
NOS-438 Alcohol and Substance-Induced Organic Mental Syndrome

(*Nos — not otherwise specified as Surgical or Medical)

MDC 21 INJURIES, POISONINGS, AND TOXIC EFFECTS OF DRUGS

S-439   Skin Grafts for Injuries
S-440   Wound Debridements for Injuries
S-441   Hand Procedures for Injuries
S-442   Other Operating Room Procedures for Injuries – Age $> = 70$ and/or CC
S-443   Other Operating Room Procedures for Injuries – Age < 70 w/o CC
M-444   Multiple Trauma – Age $> = 70$ and/or CC
M-445   Multiple Trauma – Age 18–69 w/o CC
M-446   Multiple Trauma – Age 0–17
M-447   Allergic Reactions – Age $> = 18$
M-448   Allergic Reactions – Age 0–17

M-449	Toxic Effects of Drugs – Age $\geq$ 70 and/or CC
M-450	Toxic Effects of Drugs – Age 18–69 w/o CC
M-451	Toxic Effects of Drugs – Age 0–17
M-452	Complications of Treatment – Age $\geq$ 70 and/or CC
M-453	Complications of Treatment – Age < 70 w/o CC
M-454	Other Injuries, Poisionings and Toxic Effects Diagnosis – Age $\geq$ 70 and/or CC
M-455	Other Injuries, Poisonings and Toxic Effects Diagnosis – Age < 70 w/o CC

MDC 22 BURNS: (NOS*)

NOS-456	Burns, Transferred to Another Acute Care Facility
NOS-457	Extensive Burns
S-458	Nonextensive Burns with Skin Grafts
S-459	Nonextensive Burns with Wound Debridement and Other Operating Room Procedures
M-460	Nonextensive Burns w/o Operating Room Procedures
	(*NOS — not otherwise specified as Surgical or Medical)

MDC 23 FACTORS INFLUENCING HEALTH STATUS AND OTHER CONTACTS WITH HEALTH SERVICES

S-461	Operating Room Procedures with Diagnoses of Other Contact with Health Services
M-462	Rehabilitation
M-463	Signs and Symptoms with CC
M-464	Signs and Symptoms w/o CC
M-465	Aftercare with History of Malignancy as Secondary Diagnosis
M-466	Aftercare w/o History of Malignancy as Secondary Diagnosis
M-467	Other Factors Influencing Health Status

UNGROUPABLE CASES: (NOS*)

NOS-468	Unrelated Operating Room Procedure
NOS-469	Patient Diagnosis Invalid as Discharge Diagnosis
NOS-470	Ungroupable

1

MDC 01
DISEASES AND DISORDERS
OF THE NERVOUS SYSTEM

SURGICAL GROUPINGS (8 DRGs)

Craniotomy

Spinal Procedures

Extracranial Vascular Procedures

Carpal Tunnel Release

Peripheral and Cranial Nerve Procedures

MEDICAL GROUPINGS (27 DRGs)

Spinal Disorders and Injuries

Nervous System Neoplasms

Degenerative Nervous System Disorders

Multiple Sclerosis and Cerebellar Ataxia

Cerebrovascular Disorders (specific and nonspecific)

Transient Ischemic Attacks

Cranial and Peripheral Nerve Disorders

Nervous System Infection

Viral Meningitis

Hypertensive Encephalopathy

Nontraumatic Stupor and Coma

Seizure and Headache

Traumatic Stupor and Coma

Concussion

Many conditions of the nervous system for which a patient is admitted to an acute care hospital will have long-term effects. In many cases the patient will need rehabilitation following the acute phase of the illness.

The home care needs of the patient in this MDC will depend on the type of in-hospital rehabilitation services received. The plans are designed for planning home care for patients who are deemed stable and can benefit from rehabilitation services on an intermittent basis.

MASTER HOME CARE PLANNING GUIDE
FOR DISEASES AND DISORDERS OF THE NERVOUS SYSTEM

Pattern	Assessment Factors	Plan
1. Health management deficit	How long has the patient been symptomatic? How have symptoms affected his/her management of self-care and activities of daily living? What is the prognosis for recovery of patient's decision-making ability, mentation and emotional status?	Interview patient and family along with primary caregiver to determine health management potential.
2. Alteration in nutrition secondary to chronic disease state and/or motor deficit	What are the patient's nutritional and fluid needs? Is the patient's skin status compromised from inactivity? Can the patient feed him/herself? Does the patient need adaptive equipment or specially prepared foods?	Consult with physician, dietition and occupational therapist to make plans to meet nutritional needs. See specific DRG.
3. Alteration in elimination secondary to neurological deficit	Is patient prone to incontinence of urine and/or stool? Will the patient need bladder and bowel training? Will the patient need an indwelling catheter or need to learn self-catheterization.	Establish a bowel and bladder training program early in hospital stay and instruct patient/family in the program. See specific DRG.
4. Alteration in activity and exercise pattern	Has the neurological deficit affected the patient's functional ability in any of the activities of daily living? Is the patient prone to joint contractures? Does the patient need braces or splints to carry out activities such as ambulating or feeding him/herself? Can the patient ambulate independently or does he/she need assistive devices such as canes, walkers or crutches? What was patient's prehospital functional status?	Consult with physical therapist to assess patient's balance and ambulation status. Interview patient/family about possible changes in the home to adapt to the patient's ambulation status. See specific DRG.
4a. Cognitive impairment secondary to brain involvement	What is the patient's ability to think, make decisions and comprehend surroundings? Does neurological involvement affect patient's ability at usual work or with family responsibilities?	Consult with physician and therapists to determine patient's potential for permanent changes in mentation. See specific DRG.
4b. Sensory deficit	Does the patient have a sensory deficit that will interfere with ability to communicate, ambulate or carry	In any case where a sensory deficit is suspected, a complete evaluation by a specialist

16

	out activities of daily living? Will the patient be at risk for injury because of deficit? What is the patient's vision, hearing, touch, taste and smell status?	should be done to determine the extent of the deficit and to plan therapy for correction of the deficit or changes in activities to compensate for the deficit. See specific DRG.
4c. Knowledge deficit secondary to disease process	Do the patient and family know the diagnosis and prognosis? Can the patient understand his/her illness and recognize the impact on the future?	Interview patient and family regarding disease process. Plan for counseling for patient and family to deal with overwhelming diagnosis.
5. Alteration in sleep-rest pattern	Does patient's condition change sleep and rest pattern? Does the patient need frequent rest periods? Is the patient's ability to maintain normal functioning affected by need for frequent rest periods?	See specific DRG.
6. Alteration in self-concept	Are physical changes resulting from the disease visible, or do they affect the patient's behavior or ability to function? Have these changes been gradual or have the changes appeared suddenly? Does the patient appear to be affected and depressed over changes that have occurred?	Offer counseling for patient and family. See specific DRG.
7. Alteration in role-relationship pattern	Does neurological condition affect the patient's role pattern in a spousal, parenting, working or other relationship?	Offer family counseling.
8. Potential for impaired communication	Is the patient able to communicate effectively?	Institute speech therapy as soon as possible. See specific DRG.
9. Sexual dysfunction	Does the neurological condition have an effect on the patient's ability to participate in sexual intercourse? Does the neurological condition have a permanent effect or is the condition characterized by exacerbations and remissions?	Provide information and sources of counseling for the patient and partner.
10. Potential for ineffective coping by patient and/or family	Will the patient's diagnosis and prognosis have major impact on family lifestyle? Can developmental stages continue for all family members, or will alterations need to be made by all family members? Will the family be able to meet the long-term needs of the patient from a physical, social and financial perspective?	Offer family counseling. Encourage financial counseling in conditions that will be long-term or that have a poor prognosis.
11. Spiritual distress	Does the patient and family express hope or despair? Does the patient and/or family need spiritual guidance?	Offer appropriate pastoral counseling

DRG 001

MDC 01	RW$ 3.3548	Surgical	Outlier Cutoff 39	Mean LOS 19.4

Craniotomy – Age > = 18 Except for Trauma

OPERATIVE PROCEDURES WITH POTENTIAL HOME CARE NEEDS

Ventricular shunt procedures
Pituitary gland procedures
Pineal gland procedures
Aneurysm procedures

DETAILS TO CONSIDER

Long-term needs of the patient will depend on the type of surgical procedure, the pathological condition and the outcome of the surgery itself.

POTENTIAL HOME CARE PROBLEMS

1. Health management deficit secondary to neurological involvement.

PLAN

Evaluate patient's neurological deficit, if any, and effect on ability to care for him/herself. In patients who have had a shunt procedure, instruct patient in location of shunt and possible signs and symptoms of peritonitis which may occur secondary to shunt infection. The patient should also be instructed in signs and symptoms of shunt malfunction. For patients with pituitary gland procedures, instructions in replacement therapy will be needed.

2. Alteration in self-concept with anxiety.

Inform patient and family of prognosis for disease condition and potential complications.

3. Alteration in body image secondary to removal of hair for procedure.

Assist patient in selection of wig or head cover or in ways to style hair to minimize effect of hair removal.

REFERRAL INFORMATION

Monitoring of patients after discharge will be needed, especially for malignancies, shunt procedures or aneurysm. A baseline neurological profile should be done, including patient's mentation status, ability to carry out activities of daily living and neurological deficits. A referral to hospice units for terminal patients should be made.

Patients who need hormone replacement therapy should be referred to a home care nurse for monitoring compliance. Assessing signs and symptoms of effect of therapy and, in cases where the medication is administered by injection, to assess patients's and family's ability to administer medications.

If the patient has a neurological deficit restricting mobility, assess need for physical therapy and adaptive equipment. Also assess family status and patient's care needs on a 24 hour basis.

DRG 002

MDC 01	RW$ 3.2829	Surgical	Outlier Cutoff 36	Mean LOS 15.8

Craniotomy for Trauma – Age > = 18

DIAGNOSES WITH POTENTIAL HOME CARE NEEDS

Postconcussion syndrome
Skull fracture with prolonged or deep coma

DETAILS TO CONSIDER

The needs of patients with postconcussion syndrome are usually discussed as Traumatic Brain Injury (TBI) cases. These cases require long-term intervention and may render the patient handicapped.

POTENTIAL HOME CARE PROBLEMS	PLAN
1. Health management deficit secondary to brain injury and cerebral edema.	Assess patient's cerebral status as close to discharge date as possible. Resolution of edema and return to preinjury level of functioning varies from patient to patient. Confer with physician to assess potential recovery rate, which may be dependent on length of unconsciousness and degree of memory loss. Even in mild cases a memory loss may persist for months.
1a. Coma management.	If the patient is in a deep coma, plans for total care of the patient must be made. These include nutrition, elimination, skin care, range of motion exercises and neurological stimulation.
2. Alteration in nutrition.	Alternative methods of nutrition must be considered for patients who cannot or will not eat. Tube feedings by either a nasogastric or gastrostomy tube may be needed. Instructions in tube feeding procedure must be explained to caregiver. Need for fluid balance must be stressed.
3. Alteration in elimination.	Bowel and bladder function must be monitored closely. Patient may need a training program or may need an indwelling catheter. Avoidance of constipation must be stressed.
4. Alteration in exercise.	Evaluate patient's neurological deficit and change in balance. Safety precautions may be needed for patients with balance problems.
5. Alteration in self-perception.	Patients with brain injury may have confusion which affects their ability to carry out their usual life functions. The severity of this must be evaluated, and the potential for resolution determined.
6. Potential for family stress and ineffective coping.	Evaluate impact of patient's injury and needs on the total family. Caring for a patient with brain injury can totally alter a family structure, and the potential for this must be addressed prior to discharge. Availability of respite care must be assessed.

REFERRAL INFORMATION

The decision to care for a brain-injured patient in the home must be made carefully and only after a multidisciplinary conference has been held. Persons involved include the physician, nurses, therapists, counselors, psychologists, family and home care nurse. A combination of home care and day care at a Traumatic Brain Injury Center may be selected. Referral to a rehabilitation center for a period of time with home care following is another option.

DRG 003

MDC 01	RW$ 2.9489	Surgical	Outlier Cutoff 33	Mean LOS 12.7

Craniotomy – Age 0–17

DIAGNOSES WITH POTENTIAL HOME CARE NEEDS

Postconcussion syndrome
Skull fracture with prolonged deep coma

DETAILS TO CONSIDER

See **DRG 002.**

Brain injury in the young child or adolescent becomes more complex because of the interruption in normal developmental stages. The reader is referred to pediatric texts for additional information.

DRG 004

MDC 01	RW$ 2.2452	Surgical	Outlier Cutoff 36	Mean LOS 16.0

Spinal Procedures

OPERATIVE PROCEDURES WITH POTENTIAL HOME CARE NEEDS

Percutaneous chordotomy
Spinal infusion
Myelomeningocele repair

DETAILS TO CONSIDER

The extent of long-term needs will depend on the degree of deficit following the surgery. In chordotomy the needs will depend on the underlying diagnoses. For patients under 18 the reader is referred to pediatric texts.

POTENTIAL HOME CARE PROBLEMS

1. Health management deficit secondary to underlying diagnosis and additional surgery.

2. Alteration in elimination.

3. Alteration in exercise and activity.

PLAN

Compare neurological status pre- and postsurgery and effect on patient's neurological status and health status.

Assess bowel and bladder function and evaluate need for bowel training and need for intermittent catheterization. If needed, instruct patient in self-catheterization procedure.

Assess effect of procedure on lower limb function, especially motor and sensory deficit. Patient may be paraplegic, have paresis or experience paresthesia. If any of these situations exist, physical therapy will be needed for ambulation and exercise activities.

4. Alteration in body image.

Assess impact of underlying disease and additional surgery on the patient's body image. The disease may be progressive, and the patient may need counseling for depression.

5. Alteration in sexual function.

Evaluate the effect of the surgery on the patient's sexual function and/or loss of sensation.

REFERRAL INFORMATION

Determine preadmission level of care and services that were being given. Evaluate changes needed. If pain control was a problem preadmission, it may not be a problem now. Level of self-care and additional needs because of neurological deficit need to be addressed. Refer to home care nurse for follow-up instructions in self-care or mobility problems. Equipment needed may be for self-catheterization and ambulation assistive devices.

See **DRG 009.**

DRG 005

MDC 01	RW$ 1.6780	Surgical	Outlier Cutoff 30	Mean LOS 9.8

Extracranial Vascular Procedures

OPERATIVE PROCEDURES WITH POTENTIAL HOME CARE NEEDS

Endarterectomy
Aorta-subclavian-carotid bypass

DETAILS TO CONSIDER

Patients with these procedures may have other cardiovascular diseases. The procedure usually improves the patient's health status and reduces the risk of cerebral vascular problems.

POTENTIAL HOME CARE PROBLEMS

1. Health management deficit secondary to surgery.

2. Alteration in nutrition.

PLAN

Assess patient's ability to care for self and effect of other health related conditions such as diabetes, heart disease or other peripheral vascular problems.

Instruct patient and family in prescribed dietary changes such as low cholesterol diet. Evaluate patient's financial ability to comply with dietary changes.

REFERRAL INFORMATION

If patient has other health problems, or is the caregiver to another elderly, frail person, refer to the home care nurse for home evaluation. Order special diet through Meals-on-Wheels until patient has recovered from surgery and can manage shopping and preparing meals.

DRG 006

MDC 01	RW$ 0.3993	Surgical	Outlier Cutoff 8	Mean LOS 2.6

Carpal Tunnel Release

OPERATIVE PROCEDURE WITH POTENTIAL HOME CARE NEED

Carpal tunnel release

DETAILS TO CONSIDER

This procedure is usually done as a day surgery elective procedure. Home care needs should be arranged prior to the procedure, especially if both hands will be done on the same admission. The large dressing will make it difficult for the patient to carry out activities of daily living; however, it is usually changed to a smaller dressing in a few days.

DRG 007

MDC 01	RW$ 1.0279	Surgical	Outlier Cutoff 25	Mean LOS 5.3

Peripheral and Cranial Nerve and Other Nervous System Procedures Age $\geq$ 70 and/or CC

OPERATIVE PROCEDURES WITH POTENTIAL HOME CARE NEEDS

Vagotomy
Sympathectomy

DETAILS TO CONSIDER

This procedure is done for the management of pain. The long-term needs will depend on the patient's underlying diagnosis. The effect of the comorbidity and complication should also be considered in determining long-term needs.

REFERRAL INFORMATION

Determine patient's level of care and service prehospitalization and changes in needs as a result of surgery.

| MDC 01 | RW$ 0.7239 | Surgical | Outlier Cutoff 23 | Mean LOS 4.1 |

Peripheral and Cranial Nerve and Other Nervous System Procedures Age < 70 w/o CC

See DRG 007.

| MDC 01 | RW$ 1.3958 | Medical | Outlier Cutoff 29 | Mean LOS 9.1 |

Spinal Disorders and Injuries

DIAGNOSES WITH POTENTIAL HOME CARE NEEDS

Spinal cord injury with paraplegia or quadriplegia

DETAILS TO CONSIDER

The long-term needs of patients in this group depend on many factors which include the level of injury, the type of injury, the effect of spinal shock, and the patient's developmental stage. After the initial hospitalization, the follow-up needs will vary depending on the degree of damage, stage of resolution of edema and the type of residual defect. Patients with permanent injury will need extensive rehabilitation which is usually done at a rehabilitation hospital or on a rehabilitation unit.

POTENTIAL HOME CARE PROBLEMS

1. Health management deficit secondary to permanent spinal cord injury.

2. Alteration in nutrition and potential for skin breakdown.

3. Alteration in elimination.

PLAN

Patients who suddenly become paralyzed have many health care needs which become the central focus of their existence for a long period of time. The impact of this on the patient and family must be assessed. There will need to be a major readjustment in the individual's lifestyle.

Prevention of skin breakdown over the pressure points is a goal of care that is ongoing. Special chair pads, changing position frequently and adequate nutrition needs should be arranged.

A bowel and bladder training program must be established early and maintained consistently. Bowel routine of digital stimulation, use of suppositories or other programs must be taught to the patient and family. Urine elimination by external catheter or intermittent catheterization should also be taught to patient and family.

4.	Alteration in activity and exercise.	Referral to physical therapist and occupational therapist are essential for the patient to reach maximum rehabilitation potential and for safe transfer and ambulation technique.
5.	Alteration in perceptual pattern.	Depending on the stage of resolution, the patient may have decreased or no sensations which puts the patient at risk for injury. All caregivers must be made aware of sensory problems to assist in prevention of injury.
6.	Alteration in body image.	A referral for counseling for help in adjustment to change in body image is important. Family members and significant others should be included.
7.	Alteration in role-relationship.	Plans for vocational rehabilitation should be started as soon as patient is medically stable. The role of the patient in the family may be interrupted and family counseling should be initiated early.
8.	Sexual dysfunction.	Counseling should be initiated for all patients with spinal cord injury.
9.	Potential for family stress.	Injuries of this sort have the potential for total family breakdown; thus the need to plan for respite care and long-term counseling.
10.	Alteration in value-belief pattern.	Pastoral counseling for patient and family should be offered.

REFERRAL INFORMATION

A referral for home care nurse, therapist and social worker should be made early. A multidisciplinary team conference including persons who will be doing therapy in the home should be held prior to discharge. Changes in the home to make it accessible to the patient should be evaluated prior to discharge. Short visits to the home should be made by the patient to assess which changes need to be made.

Equipment needs may include ambulation assistance devices, bathroom safety equipment, and possibly a customized wheelchair.

In the case of a discharge to home of a quadriplegic patient, occupational therapy should be consulted for adaptive equipment for eating and dressing. Follow-up medical care by neurologist, physiatrist, urologist and psychologist should be arranged in addition to vocational rehabilitation.

Nervous System Neoplasms – Age > = 70 and/or CC

DIAGNOSES WITH POTENTIAL HOME CARE NEEDS

Malignant brain neoplasms
Malignant spinal cord neoplasms
Benign neoplasm brain/spinal cord

DETAILS TO CONSIDER

Long-term care needs will depend on type and location of neoplasm and method of treatment, if any. Methods of treatment can include chemotherapy or radiation therapy or a combination. The effect of the complication or comorbidity will also need to be evaluated.

In neoplasms of the brain the patient may have central nervous system symptoms and complications such as confusion, decreased mentation and seizure activity. They may also have systemic motor and sensory defects. The patient with spinal cord neoplasms may have problems similar to those experienced by spinal cord injured patients.

POTENTIAL HOME CARE PROBLEMS

1. Health management deficit secondary to neoplasm.

2. Alteration in cognitive-perceptual pattern.

PLAN

Assess patient's ability to care for self, and assess potential effect of method of therapy on patient's ability to care for self.

Assess patient's mentation and ability to make decisions and to be responsible for self-care.

REFERRAL INFORMATION

Provide assistance in transportation for follow-up chemotherapy or radiation therapy. Refer to home care nurse to monitor patient's response to therapy and to evaluate patient's safety in the home. Patients receiving therapy for brain lesions are prone to seizures and weakness and should not be left alone during therapy. In some cases short-term admission to a skilled nursing facility may be necessary. Home care referral from the facility can also be made.

DRG 011

MDC 01   **RW$ 1.2545**   **Medical**   **Outlier Cutoff 29**   **Mean LOS 8.5**

Nervous System Neoplasms – Age < 70 w/o CC

Same as **DRG 010.**

DRG 012

MDC 01   RW$ 1.1136   Medical   Outlier Cutoff 29   Mean LOS 9.4

Degenerative Nervous System Disorders

DIAGNOSES WITH POTENTIAL HOME CARE NEEDS

Amyotrophic Sclerosis
Parkinson's Disease
Progressive Muscular Dystrophy
Myasthenia Gravis
Alzheimer's Disease

DETAILS TO CONSIDER

Hospital admissions for diagnoses in this group are usually related to a complication/exacerbation of disease with need for medical intervention.

POTENTIAL HOME CARE PROBLEMS

PLAN

1. Health management deficit secondary to changes in muscle control.

Assessment of patient's functional ability to determine self-care limits, or to assess increased need for assistance in self-care as disease progresses. The patient's decreased strength and decreased stamina will affect his/her ability to do self-care activities. An assessment of mental capabilities must be accurately done to determine patient's mental abilities to care for self.

2. Alteration in nutrition.

Assess patient's ability to feed self and swallow food. Assess need for adaptive feeding equipment and/or mechanically softened or pureed foods. Frequent meals with fluid supplements may be needed. The patient may need supervision during eating or drinking because of the danger of aspiration. A speech therapy referral is also indicated.

3. Alteration in elimination secondary to increased weakness.

The muscles needed for bowel evacuation may also be weak causing constipation. Transfer to a commode may also become more difficult.

4. Alteration in activity and exercise secondary to muscle weakness progression.

Physical and occupational therapy intervention is needed. Mechanical transfer lifts may be needed for safety of patient and caregiver. Adaptive ambulation equipment may be needed or adjusted as muscle weakness increases. Ineffective airway clearance may become a problem and lead to aspiration pneumonia. A speech therapy referral should be made.

5. Alteration in cognitive-perceptual pattern and alteration in self-concept.

In some diagnoses in this group there is an associated dementia. It is important that dementia be accurately diagnosed and that it not be confused with inability to communicate. Many patients in this group are treated as demented when they are not. The accurate assessment is vital for the patient's mental health and ability to tolerate the physical aspect of the illness.

6. Alteration in sleep-rest pattern.

The patient may have increased need for sleep and rest periods. These must be planned to maximize therapy benefit.

7. Alteration in role-relationship.

The impact of a degenerative disease on role relationships and developmental stages is overwhelming. Diseases that affect the young adult or mature adult have catastrophic effects. Counseling to assist families in coping is vital. The potential for social isolation because of increased rest needs, decreased communications ability and fear of contagion needs to be addressed. Family and friends should be instructed in the disease process and ways they can communicate effectively with the patient.

8. Alteration in value-belief pattern.

Pastoral counseling should be initiated for the patient, family and friends.

REFERRAL INFORMATION

Referral to the home care nurse, counselors, social workers, physical occupational and speech therapists will need to be made. Referral to support groups such as Multiple Sclerosis Society and Alzheimer's Support Group should also be made. Equipment needs may include ambulatory assistive devices, transfer aides, eating aids and toileting aids. An electric hospital bed may also be needed if patient's inability to swallow saliva or to clear the airway is a problem.

DRG 013

MDC 01   **RW$ 1.0150**   **Medical**   **Outlier Cutoff 29**   **Mean LOS 8.9**

Multiple Sclerosis and Cerebellar Ataxia

DIAGNOSES WITH POTENTIAL HOME CARE NEEDS

Multiple Sclerosis (MS)
Cerebellar ataxia

DETAILS TO CONSIDER

The diagnoses in this group are long-term progressive diseases. The MS patient is admitted to an acute care hospital for treatment of an acute exacerbation. It must be noted that there is a great deal of research going on related to MS and the findings may have dramatic effects on the needs of the patient.

In cerebellar ataxia there is a progression of symptoms, including ataxia, tremors and dysarthria.

POTENTIAL HOME CARE PROBLEMS

PLAN

1. Health management deficit secondary to variability of symptoms and unpredictability of disease process.

   Assess long-term needs as close to discharge as possible to better evaluate remission and stabilization status. Evaluate prehospital plan of care and determine changes that may have to be made in the plan. Evaluate ability of caregiver to manage new symptoms and progression of disease.

2. Alteration in nutrition.

   Assess patient's ability to feed self and swallow. Nutritional status should be evaluated and supplemental nutrients ordered since good nutrition is vital. Fluid intake must also be encouraged.

3. Alteration in elimination.

   Assess patient's bowel and bladder status. These functions may be affected by exacerbations and remissions and a new plan may be needed. Bowel training, indwelling catheter or intermittent catheterization may be indicated.

4. Alteration in activity-exercise secondary to loss of muscle control.

   Evaluate effect of bedrest on the patient's ability to mobilize and ambulate. Patient may need much encouragement to maintain activity because of fatigue or minor illness. Physical and occupational therapy should be carried out to plan for schedule of activity and/or assistive devices to maximize physical effort.

5. Alteration in vision.

   Evaluate vision deficit caused by progression of disease and the effect on reading, ambulating safely and self-care.

6. Alteration in sleep-rest pattern.

   Patient may be severely fatigued and need planned periods of rest. Warm weather increases fatigue factor. Patient may need to plan activities for cool periods of the day and avoid going out on warm days. This may have a major effect on the patient's and family's lifestyle.

7. Self-perception disturbance.

In some cases the patient may have a euphoric state of mind and in others there may be depression. Each patient must be evaluated and specific therapies planned dependent on the presenting symptoms. These patients need support and care throughout the disease state.

8. Alteration in role-relationship pattern.

Patients may withdraw and become socially isolated. Dysarthria may need to be managed by speech therapy and family reinforcement. In severe cases emergency call devices may need to be utilized for the patient's safety. Evaluation by a vocational counselor should be done.

9. Sexual dysfunction.

Counseling for the male patient should be done since impotence may exist. Female patients should be offered information on family planning.

10. Potential for ineffective family coping.

The effect of a progressive, degenerative illness on the family must be evaluated. The patient's developmental stage may be interrupted for a short period of time. The young adult's parenting and career status will be affected.

11. Alteration in value-belief.

The patient and family will need pastoral counseling. The feeling of hope because of research may exist. In some cases it may be so great that sitting and waiting may delay therapy. The seeking of miraculous cures at any price may affect patient's and family's lifestyle. Hope is encouraged, but therapy for existing problems should be carried out to minimize unnecessary complications.

REFERRAL INFORMATION

Refer patient to MS Society. The patient should be able to receive outpatient therapy after strength has returned to a level allowing this. For a short time after discharge the patient may need services in the home. The home environment should be evaluated for changes necessary if muscle weakness and loss of control is increasing. In most cases the patient with MS can manage at home.

For patients with cerebellar ataxia, close medical follow-up is indicated. The progression of symptoms and the increased care needs must be evaluated on an ongoing basis and plans adjusted as needs change.

DRG 014

MDC 01   **RW$ 1.3527**   **Medical**   **Outlier Cutoff 30**   **Mean LOS 9.9**

Specific Cerebrovascular Disorders Except TIA

DIAGNOSES WITH POTENTIAL HOME CARE NEEDS

Subarachnoid hemorrhage
Subdural hemorrhage
Cerebral aneurysm
Nonruptured cerebral aneurysm
Cerebral Vascular Accident (CVA)

DETAILS TO CONSIDER

Vascular problems represent a large portion of the diseases of the nervous system. This DRG represents a great number of hospital admissions. There are varied vascular problems, but the degree of brain ischemia and infarction and the location of the deficit determine the outcome of the problem. Symptoms vary according to the vasculature involved. The long-term needs will depend on the residual deficit and the possibility of extension and/or recurrence of vascular problems.

POTENTIAL HOME CARE PROBLEMS	PLAN
1. Health management deficit secondary to need for long-term, intensive rehabilitation.	Assess effect of long-term needs on patient and family lifestyle. Financial considerations must be addressed early. Assess changes in home setting that may be necessary to accommodate the patient with residual muscle weakness.
2. Alteration in nutrition.	Assess effect of muscle involvement on patient's ability to feed self and swallow. Speech therapy and occupational therapy should be consulted for assistance and adaptive equipment needs. Instructions in change in diet to decrease cholesterol intake and other medically prescribed restrictions should be given to caregiver.
3. Alteration in elimination.	Bowel and bladder training may be necessary if neural deficit involves these functions. Control of incontinence measures must be taught to patient and family.
4. Alteration in activity and exercise.	Physical and occupational therapies should be instituted as soon as patient is medically stable. The need for ambulation and transfer assistive devices should be done early so that special equipment can be used prior to discharge.
5. Alteration in sleep-rest pattern.	Patient may need periods of rest prior to therapy and meals.
6. Alteration in body image.	Counseling is indicated because of the changes in the patient's self-image. Depression and lack of motivation during therapies may hinder rehabilitation potential.

7. Alteration in role-relationship.	Patients with any aphasic disorder should receive speech therapy and counseling. The developmental stage, parenting role and vocational status must be evaluated and appropriate counseling instituted early to maximize potential.
8. Sexual dysfunction.	Potential for sexual dysfunction should be evaluated and counseling offered to the patient and significant others.
9. Potential for ineffective family coping.	The impact of the disease on the family structure should be evaluated. Financial problems may develop, structural change in the home setting may disrupt family style, inability to communicate or do self-care may direct focus of family on the patient and away from others with needs.
10. Alteration in value-belief pattern.	The "stroke" may be perceived by patient and/or family as punishment for previous behavior and may interfere with rehabilitation potential. Pastoral counseling should be offered.

REFERRAL INFORMATION

In some cases the patient may be transferred to a rehabilitation hospital or unit for intensive therapy. When the patient reaches a safe level of functioning, when 24 hour care can be arranged, and when intermittent therapy is needed, arrangements for home care should be made.

Multidisciplinary conferences should be held, including the physicians, all therapies, dietary, nursing, counselors, family and home care nurse. A trial visit to home by the patient should be made prior to discharge. Adaptive equipment and structural changes should be ready prior to discharge.

Equipment needs vary depending on the deficit and on home setting. A bed with a trapeze and side rails, a commode, bathroom safety equipment, ambulation assistive devices may all be needed.

DRG 015

MDC 01	RW$ 0.6673	Medical	Outlier Cutoff 24	Mean LOS 5.6

Transient Ischemic Attacks (TIA)

DIAGNOSIS WITH POTENTIAL HOME CARE NEEDS

Transient Ischemic Attacks (TIA)

DETAILS TO CONSIDER

A history of TIA may be indicative of potential for cerebral thrombosis.

The patient is usually admitted for investigation of the condition and to determine appropriate therapy to prevent completion of a cerebrovascular accident.

The patients treated medically for TIA are usually poor risks for surgical intervention.

POTENTIAL HOME CARE PROBLEM

Health management deficit secondary to risk for CVA.

PLAN

Assess patient's general ability to care for self and ability to follow medical regime for TIA.

REFERRAL INFORMATION

Refer the patient who is a poor surgical risk to the home care nurse for posthospital monitoring; also for education to reduce risk of CVA such as taking prescribed medications, avoiding stressful situations, restricting intake of cholesterol and getting regular medical follow-up.

DRG 016

MDC 01	RW$ 0.8592	Medical	Outlier Cutoff 27	Mean LOS 7.4

Nonspecific Cerebrovascular Disorders with CC

DIAGNOSES WITH POTENTIAL HOME CARE NEEDS

Encephalopathy
Cerebral atherosclerosis
Cerebral vascular disease

DETAILS TO CONSIDER

Causes of encephalopathy vary greatly. In these cases there is no detectable lesion causing the symptoms, and it is assumed to be a subcellular level condition. It may be caused by a chemical toxic agent or by a nutritional deficiency.

The long-term needs will depend on the underlying cause, the effect of the pathology on the patient's mentation and ability to carry out activities of daily living, and the complication or comorbidity.

POTENTIAL HOME CARE PROBLEM

Health management deficit secondary to central nervous system involvement.

PLAN

Evaluate patient's ability to care for self, or in some cases to care for others. Assess patient's response to therapy and potential for compliance with regime.

REFERRAL INFORMATION

Refer any patient with an encephalopathy who will need to follow a medical regime including medications, nutritional changes or changes in lifestyle. During hospitalization the patient's confusion or decreased mental capabilities may make retention of information impossible. Reinforcement of medical plan is necessary.

DRG 017

MDC 01	RW$ 0.8392	Medical	Outlier Cutoff 27	Mean LOS 7.2

Nonspecific Cerebrovascular Disorders w/o CC

DIAGNOSES WITH POTENTIAL HOME CARE NEEDS

Encephalopathy
Cerebral atherosclerosis
Cerebral vascular disease

See **DRG 016.**

DRG 018

MDC 01	RW$ 0.7915	Medical	Outlier Cutoff 27	Mean LOS 6.6

Cranial and Peripheral Nerve Disorders – Age $> = 70$ and/or CC

DIAGNOSES WITH POTENTIAL HOME CARE NEEDS

Neuropathy in diabetes
Alcoholic polyneuropathy

DETAILS TO CONSIDER

The long-term needs will depend on the underlying diagnosis. Admissions in this group are related to complications to other diseases.

See **DRG 294** and **295** for information on diabetes. Refer to texts on alcoholism for additional information.

POTENTIAL HOME CARE PROBLEM

Health management deficit secondary to complication of other diagnosis.

PLAN

Assess impact of deficit on patient's ability to care for self, especially in vision problems or of legs and feet affecting ambulation.

REFERRAL INFORMATION

Patient may be known to a home health agency because of diagnosis. New information about the patient's change in self-care ability or need for additional medical care should be communicated.

DRG 019

MDC 01	RW$ 0.6975	Medical	Outlier Cutoff 26	Mean LOS 5.7

Cranial and Peripheral Nerve Disorders – Age < 70 w/o CC

See **DRG 018.**

DRG 020

MDC 01	RW$ 1.3141	Medical	Outlier Cutoff 28	Mean LOS 7.6

Nervous System Infection Except Viral Meningitis

DIAGNOSES WITH POTENTIAL HOME CARE NEEDS

Meningitis
Encephalitis

DETAILS TO CONSIDER

The course of the disease will depend on the causative agent and the effectiveness of therapy. Even with adequate and early treatment infection may gradually resolve, but residual changes may occur. In severe cases residual changes may lead to hydrocephalus, dementia, paralysis, coma or vision changes.

If diagnosed and managed early the prognosis for complete recovery is good.

POTENTIAL HOME CARE PROBLEM

Health management deficit secondary to need for long-term follow-up.

PLAN

Assess patient's or family's ability to get medical follow-up. Instruct in signs and symptoms of later complications of disease.

REFERRAL INFORMATION

Refer to the home care nurse any patient who is suspect for late effects of disease, or who may have health management needs at the time of discharge. The disease is reportable and contacts should be followed for possible disease.

Viral Meningitis

DIAGNOSIS WITH POTENTIAL HOME CARE NEEDS

Viral Meningitis

DETAILS TO CONSIDER

See **DRG 020.**

Residual effects lasting a year or more may include weakness, muscle spasm, insomnia and personality changes.

POTENTIAL HOME CARE PROBLEMS

1. Health management deficit secondary to residual effects.

2. Alteration in activity and exercise.

3. Alteration in sleep-rest pattern.

4. Potential for ineffective family coping.

PLAN

Assess severity of residual effect on patient's ability to care for self, or of caregiver's ability to manage patient.

Physical therapy should be taught for muscle strengthening and for treatment for muscle spasms.

Instruct patient and family in ways to cope with insomnia such as avoiding stimulants (alcohol and caffeine) in the evening, not taking late afternoon or evening naps; plan purposeful relaxing activities if patient cannot sleep at night.

Personality changes may exhibit as behavior disorder or as hostile-aggressive behavior. Instruct family in ways to manage behavior without disruption of the family structure. Counseling and medical follow-up is needed.

DRG 022

Hypertensive Encephalopathy

DIAGNOSES WITH POTENTIAL HOME CARE NEEDS

Compression of brain
Cerebral edema

DETAILS TO CONSIDER

These diagnoses are of an acute nature. The long-term needs will depend on the degree of brain damage and the underlying cause. The progression of this pathology may, in some cases, lead to a clinical situation referred to as "brain death."

POTENTIAL HOME CARE PROBLEM

Health management deficit secondary to unknown outcome of condition.

PLAN

a. Assessment of the patient's ability to participate in self-care must be done.
b. If patient may be classified as brain dead, the hospital protocol for such cases should be followed.

REFERRAL INFORMATION

Referral to home health nurse to evaluate patient's abilities to carry out activities of daily living and to monitor improvement of neurological status. If patient is brain dead, referral for requesting organ donation as outlined in hospital protocol should be initiated early.

DRG 023

Nontraumatic Stupor and Coma

DIAGNOSES WITH POTENTIAL HOME CARE NEEDS

Compression of brain
Cerebral edema

DETAILS TO CONSIDER

Stupor and coma are usually due to organic cerebral dysfunction; thus the long-term needs will depend on the underlying cause and any residual deficit.

See **DRG 022.**

| MDC 01 | RW$ 0.7279 | Medical | Outlier Cutoff 26 | Mean LOS 5.6 |

Seizure and Headache – Age > = 70 and/or CC

DIAGNOSES WITH POTENTIAL HOME CARE NEEDS

Epilepsy
Migraine headaches
Convulsions
Headache

DETAILS TO CONSIDER

Symptoms of the central nervous system in this group may have a long-term effect on the patient. The conditions are usually of a chronic nature and managed medically.

POTENTIAL HOME CARE PROBLEMS

PLAN

1. Health care deficit secondary to chronic condition and need for ongoing medical management.

Instruct patient and family in disease process and behavior to control effect of symptoms. Education regarding illness and fact that most patients can lead a normal life should be done for patient and family.

1a. Potential for noncompliance.

Assess the ability of the patient and family to understand the medication regime and the modification in behavior needed to control symptoms.

REFERRAL INFORMATION

If symptoms cause the patient to be at risk in some environments, vocational counseling may be necessary. Arrangements for medical follow-up must be made. If there is a potential for noncompliance, refer to the home health nurse for monitoring safety of the patient in the home.

| MDC 01 | RW$ 0.6392 | Medical | Outlier Cutoff 25 | Mean LOS 4.9 |

Seizure and Headache – Age 18–69 w/o CC

See **DRG 024.**

DRG 026

MDC 01	RW$ 0.4349	Medical	Outlier Cutoff 13	Mean LOS 3.3

Seizure and Headache – Age 0–17

See **DRG 024.**

DETAILS TO CONSIDER

The reader is encouraged to consult pediatric references for additional information.

DRG 027

MDC 01	RW$ 1.1368	Medical	Outlier Cutoff 24	Mean LOS 4.1

Traumatic Stupor and Coma, Coma > 1 hour

DIAGNOSES WITH POTENTIAL HOME CARE NEEDS

Skull fracture
Brain hemorrhage
Laceration or contusion with coma

DETAILS TO CONSIDER

See **DRG 002** and **023.**

In the conditions in this group, the patient does not undergo craniotomy. The patient may be admitted for observation following an episode of unconsciousness for longer than one hour, or the patient may be unconscious at the time of admission and wake up shortly after. Long-term needs will depend on the residual effect of the trauma including weakness, loss of function or loss of memory.

| MDC 01 | RW$ 1.0701 | Medical | Outlier Cutoff 26 | Mean LOS 5.9 |

Traumatic Stupor and Coma, Coma < 1 hr
Age > = 70 and/or CC

DIAGNOSES WITH POTENTIAL HOME CARE NEEDS

Skull fracture
Brain hemorrhage
Laceration or contusion with coma

DETAILS TO CONSIDER

The long-term effects will depend on the residual effect of the trauma and on the comorbidity and/or complication.

See **DRGs 002, 023** and **027**.

| MDC 01 | RW$ 0.7175 | Medical | Outlier Cutoff 24 | Mean LOS 3.8 |

Traumatic Stupor and Coma,
Coma < 1 hr – Age 18–69 w/o CC

Same as **DRG 028**.

| MDC 01 | RW$ 0.3576 | Medical | Outlier Cutoff 8 | Mean LOS 2.0 |

Traumatic Stupor and Coma,
Coma < 1 hr – Age 0–17

Same as **DRG 027**.

DETAILS TO CONSIDER

The reader is referred to pediatric texts for additional information.

DRG 031

MDC 01	RW$ 0.6051	Medical	Outlier Cutoff 25	Mean LOS 4.6

Concussion – Age > = 70 and/or CC

DIAGNOSIS WITH POTENTIAL HOME CARE NEEDS

Concussion

DETAILS TO CONSIDER

Patients with concussion are usually admitted to the hospital for observation or because of a comorbidity which increases the patient's risk of serious side effects. The usual course of recovery for persons who have had a concussion is a return to preinjury level of functioning within a short time. The duration of posttrauma amnesia may last for several months.

POTENTIAL HOME CARE PROBLEMS

1. Health management deficit secondary to head injury and amnesia.

2. Alteration in socialization.

PLAN

Evaluate the patient's ability to care for self, especially in the frail elderly and in patients with significant comorbidity. If the concussion was related to an intentional injury, the patient may need counseling.

Follow-up monitoring should be done. The elderly patient may become fearful and become unable to manage activities of daily living that require leaving home.

REFERRAL INFORMATION

Referral to the home care nurse for follow-up monitoring of home management should be done. Contact local police department and social services department to inform them of the discharge of the at-risk patient.

DRG 032

MDC 01	RW$ 0.4519	Medical	Outlier Cutoff 19	Mean LOS 3.3

Concussion – Age 18–69 w/o CC

Same as **DRG 031.**

MDC 01   RW$ 0.2483   Medical   Outlier Cutoff 5   Mean LOS 1.6

Concussion – Age 0–17

Same as **DRG 031**.

DETAILS TO CONSIDER

The reader is referred to pediatric texts for additional information.

MDC 01   RW$ 0.9927   Medical   Outlier Cutoff 27   Mean LOS 7.1

Other Disorders of Nervous System
Age > = 70 and/or CC

DIAGNOSES WITH POTENTIAL HOME CARE NEEDS

Tics
Tremors
Insomnia with sleep apnea

DETAILS TO CONSIDER

The long-term needs will depend on the underlying cause of the problem, if known, and the effect on the patient's ability to carry out activities of daily living.

POTENTIAL HOME CARE PROBLEMS

1. Health management deficit secondary to tremor.

2. Alteration in sleep-rest pattern secondary to sleep apnea.

PLAN

Assess patient's ability to carry out activities of daily living, drive a car or remain in usual employment.

Assess need for evaluation by ear, nose and throat specialist for surgical intervention. Assess patient's use of alcohol or hypnotic drugs that may relate to apneic periods. Determine need for monitoring and oxygen. Instruct patient and family in regime planned to control apnea.

REFERRAL INFORMATION

Arrangements for follow-up medical care and instructions in use of monitoring equipment (if used) should be done prior to discharge.

DRG 035

Other Disorders of Nervous System
Age < 70 w/o CC

Same as **DRG 034.**

DETAILS TO CONSIDER

See **DRG 034.**

Sleep apnea in the neonate is a serious problem which can be controlled by apnea monitors. The reader is referred to pediatric texts for additional information.

2 MDC 02
DISEASES AND DISORDERS OF THE EYE

SURGICAL GROUPINGS (7 DRGs)

Retinal, Orbital, Primary and Lens Procedures

Extraocular Procedures

Intraocular Procedures

MEDICAL GROUPINGS (6 DRGs)

Hyphema

Acute Eye Infection

Neurological Eye Disorders

MASTER HOME CARE PLANNING GUIDE
FOR CONDITIONS OF THE EYE

Pattern	Assessment Factors	Plan
1. Alteration in vision	History of vision problems, including blurring, appearance of "floating" objects, pain, trauma and infection. Family history of conditions such as glaucoma very important.	Documents patient's response, especially regarding visual field aspects. These symptoms are often transitory.
2. Potential for alteration in self-image	Conditions of the eye and orbit are obvious and have major impact on appearance. Patient's ability to handle change needs to be assessed.	If condition results in permanent change in appearance, psychological counseling may be needed.
3. Alteration in role-relationship	If the patient's eye condition will result in diminution of vision or blindness, the effect on changes in role regarding family, spouse, children and on the job duties must be assessed.	The LOS for MDC 02 ranges up to 6.5 days. Early detection by hospital staff of alteration in lifestyle and referral to appropriate sources are vital. Referrals to Family Counseling Agencies and agencies providing services to the blind are essential. The patient may not be ready for contact because of the severity of the potential handicap, but the contact to the agency should be made early.
4. Alteration in coping-stress pattern	Vision problems may be yet another complication for the diabetic and will have an impact on patient's ability to do self-care. Hospitalization may be an emergency and patient will be ill-prepared to cope. The condition may be from trauma and patient may experience a great deal of fear regarding the outcome. Determine from physician the potential for long-term visual deficit.	Allow patient time to verbalize feelings and help patient plan a method to deal with present situation. Include family member or significant other person in discussion with the patient.
5. Alteration in activity-exercise pattern	Interruption in pattern may be necessary to protect the delicate structure of the eye, or because patient's vision will be affected. Assess patient's awareness of potential changes in peripheral vision and depth perception when one eye is patched.	Be sure patient understands reason for necessary changes in activity. Consult with surgeon to determine activity restrictions indicated. Each procedure has specific follow-up instructions regarding lifting, bending and other activities. Driving and operation of other machinery may be contraindicated for the patient's safety.

Retinal Procedures

OPERATIVE PROCEDURES WITH POTENTIAL HOME CARE NEEDS

Surgical procedures to correct a detached retina, torn retina or a retina with a hole.

DETAILS TO CONSIDER

Cause of detachment will have an effect on the prognosis. The detachment may be the cause for hospitalization but there may be other serious diagnoses. Diabetes may be a factor in detachment. By the date of discharge most patient's care will be self-care and most can resume normal activity in 3–6 weeks.

POTENTIAL HOME CARE PROBLEMS

PLAN

1. Potential reoccurrence of detachment.

Possibility of future detachment is great; therefore the patient and family should be made aware of the classic symptoms of detachment. These include floating spots or progression of a visual field defect. Patient should be instructed to seek medical treatment immediately if symptoms occur.

2. Alteration in vision.

Determine what the patient's potential postoperative vision status will be compared to the predetachment vision. The prognosis for the diabetic patient may be unknown. If vision has decreased, evaluate patient's potential self-care problems, especially if self-administering insulin. Also assess for safety in ambulation in the home environment.

REFERRAL INFORMATION

If condition is uncomplicated there will be no referral needs. By the date of discharge most patients will be following self-care and most can resume normal activity in 3–6 weeks. If detachment is related to other conditions such as diabetes, referral for follow-up may be indicated. If there are potential family problems refer to **Social Services.**

DRG 037

Orbital Procedures

OPERATIVE PROCEDURES WITH POTENTIAL HOME CARE NEEDS

Orbitotomy
Eye evisceration
Eyeball enucleation
Orbital exenteration
Remove ocular implant
Excision orbital lesion

DETAILS TO CONSIDER

The surgical approach to surgeries in this DRG is relatively direct; hence a relatively short length of stay. There is usually little impact on the patient's ability to carry out activities of daily living unless both eyes are involved or there is vision impairment in the other eye.

POTENTIAL HOME CARE PROBLEM

Alteration in depth perception secondary to loss of one eye.

PLAN

Make patient aware of change in vision that may affect driving or operation of other machinery.

REFERRAL INFORMATION

Determine patient's visual status and, if patient will be blind, refer to **Social Services** for follow-up.

DRG 038

Primary Iris Procedures

OPERATIVE PROCEDURES WITH POTENTIAL HOME CARE NEEDS

Iridotomy
Glaucoma procedure and release of adhesions of the iris to the cornea (goniosynechiae)

DETAILS TO CONSIDER

Glaucoma usually affects both eyes and if left untreated can cause blindness. The purpose of the surgical procedure in the treatment of glaucoma is to create a new channel through which aqueous humor can leave the eye, thus reducing the intraocular pressure.

POTENTIAL HOME CARE PROBLEMS

1. Alteration in lifestyle to protect vision.

2. Anxiety related to second eye surgery.

REFERRAL INFORMATION

See **Master Care Plan.**

PLAN

Patient should attempt to avoid activities which increase ocular pressure such as emotional stress or heavy exertion. Also avoidance of wearing tight clothing around the neck or waist. Upper respiratory infections resulting in coughing should be treated early with cough preparations.

Allow patient an opportunity to verbalize feelings. If procedure is done on same admission, expected LOS will be altered.

DRG 039

| MDC 02 | RW$ 0.5010 | Surgical | Outlier Cutoff 6 | Mean LOS 2.8 |

Lens Procedures

OPERATIVE PROCEDURES WITH POTENTIAL HOME CARE NEEDS

Procedures to treat cataracts

DETAILS TO CONSIDER

There are many types of procedures to remove the opaque lens of the cataract patient. The cataract results from the aging process, diabetes, eye infection, or rarely from chemicals or physical elements. Cataracts are painless conditions which lead to distorted or blurred vision. Surgery must be done at a specific time so the patient may have been anticipating surgery for a period of time. A lens, to replace the removed opaque lens, can be implanted into the eye to correct the vision of some patients.

POTENTIAL HOME CARE PROBLEMS

See **Master Care Plan.**

DRG 040

Extraocular Procedures Except Orbit – Age > = 18

OPERATIVE PROCEDURES WITH POTENTIAL HOME CARE PROBLEMS

Surgical procedures in this group are performed on structures of the eye such as eyelid, muscles, lacrimal gland, conjunctiva and blood vessels.

Corneal surgery is also included in this extraocular grouping because the eyeball is not entered, but the surgery is performed on the outside.

Keratoplasty or corneal transplant is indicated.

DETAILS TO CONSIDER

Potential for vision impairment is not as great in these conditions. Improvement in vision is often the goal of treatment. Some procedures are done for cosmetic effect or for neurological conditions which result in ptosis (drooping of the lids).

POTENTIAL HOME CARE PROBLEM

Alteration in activity pattern.

PLAN

Instruct patient in details of activity restriction, especially following corneal surgery. Eye rest may be indicated, in which case both eyes should be patched. Patients should wear protective shield for extended time, sometimes up to 6 weeks. Lifting of objects of greater than 5 lbs., straining at stool or bending with head in dependent position should be avoided.

MDC 02   RW$ 0.3695   Surgical   Outlier Cutoff 4   Mean LOS 1.6

Extraocular Procedures Except Orbit – Age 0–17

OPERATIVE PROCEDURES WITH POTENTIAL HOME CARE NEEDS

See **DRG 040.**

DETAILS TO CONSIDER

Surgery on eye muscles can be done as early as 9–24 months with good results.

Treatment of congenital ptosis is performed around the age of 3–4 years. Surgery may be done earlier if ptosis is severe and blocks the pupil. If left untreated, visual development may be impaired.

POTENTIAL HOME CARE PROBLEM	PLAN
Alteration in parenting due to hospitalization of the child.	Assess potential parenting problems if child has a congenital defect or has problems related to trauma.

REFERRAL INFORMATION

Assure plans for follow-up care for child. Frequently surgery on the eye is done at specialty hospitals and the family may be far from home.

MDC 02   RW$ 0.5906   Surgical   Outlier Cutoff 12   Mean LOS 3.8

Intraocular Procedures Except Retina, Lens and Iris

OPERATIVE PROCEDURES WITH POTENTIAL HOME CARE NEEDS

Procedures in this group are related to trauma to the eyeball itself; glaucoma procedures involving the structures of the eye to allow fluid to drain, procedures in which the fluid of the eye is involved.

DETAILS TO CONSIDER

Trauma to the eyeball is serious and may lead to infection and blindness.

See **Master Care Plan** and **DRG 038.**

DRG 043

MDC 02	RW$ 0.3828	Medical	Outlier Cutoff 12	Mean LOS 4.2

Hyphema

PRINCIPAL DIAGNOSIS WITH POTENTIAL HOME CARE NEEDS

Hyphema is a condition characterized by hemorrhage within the anterior chamber of the eye.

DETAILS TO CONSIDER

This is a serious injury and secondary bleeding is frequent and occurs usually within 6 days after the primary bleed.

POTENTIAL HOME CARE PROBLEMS	PLAN
1. Potential permanent changes in vision and corneal staining.	Reinforce need for follow-up vision care.
2. Sensory deprivation due to binocular patches.	If patient becomes agitated by binocular patch, contact physician regarding possible monocular patching.

REFERRAL INFORMATION

Patients with hyphema should be examined for development of glaucoma. If patient is black, advise for sickle-cell screening.

DRG 044

MDC 02	RW$ 0.6298	Medical	Outlier Cutoff 22	Mean LOS 6.5

Acute Major Eye Infections

DETAILS TO CONSIDER

Major eye infections can lead to blindness. Crossover of infection to unaffected eye must be vigorously avoided.

See **Master Care Plan.**

POTENTIAL HOME CARE PROBLEM	PLAN
Potential for reinfection or crossover infection.	Instruct patient in good hygiene habits such as handwashing, keeping hands away from eyes, and using separate towel and wash cloth. If patient is young, evaluation of siblings and schoolmates may be indicated.

MDC 02   RW$ 0.5641   **Medical**   **Outlier Cutoff 18**   **Mean LOS 4.3**

Neurological Eye Disorders

PRINCIPAL DIAGNOSIS WITH POTENTIAL HOME CARE NEEDS

Conditions in this group are eye disorders associated with nerve pathways and other neurological conditions. Half of the cranial nerves are associated with the eye, its function and movement. Signs and symptoms associated with the eye are frequently caused by other neurological disorders.

REFERRAL INFORMATION

Referral needs are varied in this DRG depending on the underlying etiology.

Refer to specific DRGs related to patient's diagnosis.

MDC 02   RW$ 0.5964   **Medical**   **Outlier Cutoff 23**   **Mean LOS 4.1**

Other Disorders of the Eye – Age $\geq$ 18 with CC

PRINCIPAL DIAGNOSES WITH POTENTIAL HOME CARE NEEDS

TB of the eye
Trachoma
Syphilitic optic atrophy
Gonococcal infection
Malignancy of eyelid and related organs
Pigment retina dystrophy
Burns

DETAILS TO CONSIDER

Conditions in this group can lead to blindness. Treatment depends on cause of problem. Complications can include general poor health and hygiene because of poor socioeconomic status. Burns of the eyes can also be associated with respiratory burns or chemical burns of eyelids with resultant scarring and retracting.

See **Master Care Plan.**

DRG 047

MDC 02	RW$ 0.5064	Medical	Outlier Cutoff 12	Mean LOS 3.0

Other Disorders of the Eye – Age > = 18 w/o CC

See **DRG 046.**

DRG 048

MDC 02	RW$ 0.4060	Medical	Outlier Cutoff 13	Mean LOS 2.9

Other Disorders of the Eye – Age 0–17

See **DRGs 41, 46** and **47.**

3 MDC 03
DISEASES AND DISORDERS OF THE EAR, NOSE AND THROAT

SURGICAL GROUPINGS (15 DRGs)

Major Head and Neck Procedures

Sialoadenectomy

Salivary Gland Procedures

Cleft Lip and Palate Repair

Sinus and Mastoid Procedures

Rhinoplasty

Tonsillectomy and Adenoidectomy Procedures

Tonsillectomy and/or Adenoidectomy

Myringotomy

MEDICAL GROUPINGS (11 DRGs)

Ear, Nose and Throat Malignancy

Dysequilibrium

Epistaxis

Epiglottitis

Otitis Media and Upper Respiratory Infection

Laryngotracheitis

Nasal Trauma and Deformity

Other Diagnoses

In this MDC the diagnoses are grouped because of anatomical relationship. Three distinct systems are ivolved: the ear, the nose, and the mouth and throat. Because of this there will be three separate Master Care Plans for this MDC.

MASTER HOME CARE PLANNING GUIDE
FOR CONDITIONS OF THE EAR

Pattern	Assessment Factors	Plan
1. Health management deficit secondary to impaired hearing	Will the patient's hearing affect the ability to communicate over the phone? Will the patient be able to hear someone speaking? Is the patient responsible for the care of others such as young children or another disabled person? Will a decreased ability to hear affect the patient's ability to drive or work? Will the patient have improved hearing thereby decreasing previous restrictions in lifestyle?	Refer to an audiologist. Investigate alternative methods of calling for help. Encourage patient and family to notify neighbors and local police and fire department of patient's decreased ability to hear.
1a. Impaired balance	Will the patient's balance problems affect the ability to drive or work? Does the patient have side effects of poor balance such as nausea, dizziness or irritability.	Instruct patient in medical regime and safety measures during periods of imbalance.
1b. Potential for recurrent infections	Has the patient had recurrent ear infections and recurrent upper respiratory tract infections?	Instruct patient and family of need to complete antibiotic therapy, to avoid contact with persons with respiratory illnesses and to stop smoking and avoid areas where people are smoking. Instruct patient in oral hygiene and to not hold one nostril closed when blowing nose. This will prevent back pressure and possible forcing of secretions into sinuses. Instruct patient to seek and follow physician recommendations regarding swimming and other possible activity restrictions.

MASTER HOME CARE PLANNING GUIDE
FOR CONDITIONS OF THE NOSE (AND SINUSES)

Pattern	Assessment Factors	Plan
1. Health management	Length of stay is relatively short; thus arrangements must be made for follow-up care.	Instruct patient in signs and symptoms of complications. Verify plans for medical follow-up.
1a. Alteration in airway clearance	Will patient be able to maintain a clear airway? Can patient chew food and swallow fluids without the danger of aspiration.	Instruct patient to avoid contact with persons who have upper respiratory infections. Instruct patient in oral hygiene. Instruct patient to eat soft foods, take small mouthfuls of food and small sips of liquid.

MASTER HOME CARE PLANNING GUIDE
FOR CONDITIONS OF THE MOUTH AND THROAT

Pattern	Assessment Factors	Plan
1. Health management deficit	What effect does disease or surgical procedure have on patient's ability to care for self, or on caregiver? What is the permanent effect on the patient's ability to carry out activities of daily living?	Instruct patient and family in all procedures, including mouth care, wound care and airway clearance. See specific DRG.
2. Alteration in nutrition	Does the surgical procedure affect the patient's ability to eat normally? Does the disease interrupt normal digestive functions?	See specific DRG. Instruct patient and family in method selected for providing nutrition.
3. Alteration in elimination	Does the necessary alteration in nutrition affect bowel elimination? Does the patient have a potential for diarrhea or constipation?	Instruct patient in expected changes in elimination, diet modifications to control problems and when to report problems to the physician.
4. Alteration in activity such as ineffective airway clearance.	Will the patient be able to maintain a clear airway by normal methods or will he/she need a mechanical suction device? Is there a potential for aspiration? Does the patient have a productive cough?	Instruct patient in need to clear airway and throat of mucus secretions. Advise and encourage the patient who smokes to **STOP.** Involve speech therapy if patient has an airway clearance or swallowing problem. See specific DRG.
4a. Self-care deficit	Will the patient be able to manage self-care such as airway clearance, nutritional procedure and wound care? Can the patient communicate over the phone, thereby allowing him/her to be left alone? Will the patient be able to swallow prescribed medications?	Instruct patient and family in all procedures. See specific DRG.

5.	Pain management problems	If the patient is experiencing pain will he/she be able to take oral medications? Will pain medication suppress coughing or depress respirations, thus affecting the patient's ability to clear the airway?	Instruct patient in effect of pain medication and alternative methods of pain control such as rest or diversional activities.
6.	Alteration in self-concept	Will the surgery change the appearance of the patient? Will the patient's body image be altered as a result of the surgery?	Offer counseling for patients who have a change in physical appearance.
7.	Alteration in role-relationship secondary to impaired verbal communications	Will the patient be able to speak normally after healing has taken place? Will he/she need a permanent device for speech? Can the patient learn esophageal speech?	Refer to speech therapist.

DRG 049

MDC 03	RW$ 2.5270	Surgical	Outlier Cutoff 34	Mean LOS 13.6

Major Head and Neck Procedures

OPERATIVE PROCEDURES WITH POTENTIAL HOME CARE NEEDS

Glossectomy — partial, complete and radical
Laryngectomy — partial, complete and radical
Radical neck dissection
Mandibulectomy

DETAILS TO CONSIDER

See **Master Care Plan** for mouth and throat.

Long-term needs will depend on underlying disease. If it is a malignancy and is treated early, the likelihood of a cure is great.

POTENTIAL HOME CARE PROBLEMS

1. Health management deficit secondary to complex care.

2. Alteration in nutrition.

PLAN

Instruct patient and family in all aspects of care including airway clearance, wound care, nutrition, medication regime and plans for restoration of speech.

If patient has a tube for feeding, instruct patient and family in the following points:
- where the tube goes: e.g. is it a nasogastric tube, an esophageal tube, or a gastrostomy tube?
- what is the method of feeding, such as gravity feed, a feeding pump, an 8-hour nighttime program or 24-hour program?
- what is the best source of nutrition, such as blenderized food or commercially prepared product?
- what is the name and number of the company providing the supplies for use in the home.

3. Alteration in airway clearance.

Instruct patient in self-suctioning techniques. Instruct patient and family in care of the tracheostomy or laryngectomy tube and surrounding skin. Consult with a respiratory therapist for the regime for pulmonary toileting.

REFERRAL INFORMATION

Referral for home care services for patients in this DRG should be made. Any patient with nutritional problems, airway clearance problems or tracheostomy or laryngectomy tube and wound care problems needs to have follow-up care. Referral for speech therapy should be made prior to discharge.

Consideration of equipment needs should include whether patient will need to sleep with head of bed elevated or will need to change positions frequently or quickly. If so, a hospital bed will be needed. The need for a suction machine and catheters, humidifying apparatus and an emergency call system should be considered.

DRG 050

MDC 03	RW$ 0.7160	Surgical	Outlier Cutoff 14	Mean LOS 4.6

Sialoadenectomy

OPERATIVE PROCEDURES WITH POTENTIAL HOME CARE NEEDS

Sialoadenectomy (excision of a salivary gland)

DETAILS TO CONSIDER

The long-term needs will depend on the prognosis for the condition. In most cases the patient will be able to carry out self-care.

POTENTIAL HOME CARE PROBLEMS

1. Alteration in activity pattern.

2. Potential alteration in sensations secondary to surgical procedure.

PLAN

Instruct patient in need for and procedure for oral hygiene.

Instruct patient that some numbness of the ear may occur. Verify with the physician what the status of the nerves are and the potential for recovery of sensation over the course of a year.

DRG 051

MDC 03	RW$ 0.6702	Surgical	Outlier Cutoff 15	Mean LOS 4.2

Salivary Gland Procedures Except Sialoadenectomy

OPERATIVE PROCEDURES WITH POTENTIAL HOME CARE NEEDS

Marsupialization of cysts
Fistula closure

Refer to **DRG 050.**

DRG 052

MDC 03	RW$ 0.6488	Surgical	Outlier Cutoff 11	Mean LOS 3.8

Cleft Lip and Palate Repair

DETAILS TO CONSIDER

This procedure is usually done on the young child. The reader is referred to pediatric texts for more information.

DRG 053

MDC 03	RW$ 0.5895	Surgical	Outlier Cutoff 11	Mean LOS 3.5

Sinus and Mastoid Procedures – Age > = 18

OPERATIVE PROCEDURES WITH POTENTIAL HOME CARE NEEDS

Mastoidectomy
Frontal sinusotomy
Sinusectomy
Ethmoidectomy
Sphenoidectomy
Nasal sinus fistula closure

DETAILS TO CONSIDER

The long-term needs will depend on the underlying disease. If the underlying diagnosis is one of a malignancy, the patient will need long-term follow-up. This site may be a primary site or a metastasis. Because of the proximity of the disease to the brain, the patient should be followed for neurological complications.

DRG 054

MDC 03	RW$ 0.6961	Surgical	Outlier Cutoff 11	Mean LOS 3.2

Sinus and Mastoid Procedures – Age 0–17

Same as **DRG 053**.

The reader is referred to pediatric texts for further information.

| MDC 03 | RW$ 0.4153 | Surgical | Outlier Cutoff 7 | Mean LOS 2.5 |

Miscellaneous Ear, Nose and Throat Procedures

OPERATIVE PROCEDURES WITH POTENTIAL HOME CARE NEEDS

Myringoplasty
Tympanoplasty
Inner ear fenestration

DETAILS TO CONSIDER

These procedures are designed to restore hearing in patients. They are elective procedures done on a noninfected ear.

| MDC 03 | RW$ 0.4144 | Surgical | Outlier Cutoff 8 | Mean LOS 2.8 |

Rhinoplasty

OPERATIVE PROCEDURES WITH POTENTIAL HOME CARE NEEDS

Total reconstruction
Augmentation

DETAILS TO CONSIDER

These are elective procedures done for cosmetic reasons or for an obstructed nasal passage.

DRG 057

Tonsil and Adenoid Procedures Except Tonsillectomy and/or Adenoidectomy – Age > = 18

OPERATIVE PROCEDURES WITH POTENTIAL HOME CARE NEEDS

ID peritonsillar abscess
Excision tonsil tag
Biopsy
Hemorrhage control post T and A

DETAILS TO CONSIDER

This is usually an acute episode of illness that will be limited in duration.

POTENTIAL HOME CARE PROBLEMS	PLAN
1. Health management deficit.	Teach importance of oral hygiene, frequent rinsing of mouth and avoidance of astringent mouthwash. Brush teeth 3 times a day. Teach that hemorrhage may occur up to 8 days after the procedure when sutures are absorbed. Avoid people with upper respiratory infections. Avoid smoking.
2. Alteration in nutrition to avoid irritation to operative site.	Provide patient/family with list of foods allowed. Cool liquids. Progress to soft diet as tolerated. Avoid hot, spicy foods, raw vegetables, citrus juices, toast and crackers. Chew foods well and swallow slowly. Avoid sucking on straws.
3. Pain control.	Teach importance of taking prescribed medications. Avoid aspirin because of blood coagulation interference. Take cool liquids for comfort.
4. Alteration in elimination.	Avoid straining during bowel movements. The patient may need a mild laxative. Stool may be tarry due to swallowed blood.
5. Alteration in activity/exercise pattern.	Teach patient and family the importance of limited activity, no heavy lifting, no vigorous exercise; avoid sneezing, coughing or clearing of throat.

MDC 03	RW$ 0.3130	Surgical	Outlier Cutoff 3	Mean LOS 1.5

Tonsil and Adenoid Procedures Except Tonsillectomy and/or Adenoidectomy – Age 0–17

See **DRG 057.**

DETAILS TO CONSIDER

The reader is referred to pediatric texts for additional information.

MDC 03	RW$ 0.3147	Surgical	Outlier Cutoff 4	Mean LOS 2.0

Tonsillectomy and/or Adenoidectomy – Age > = 18

OPERATIVE PROCEDURES WITH POTENTIAL HOME CARE NEEDS

Tonsillectomy
T and A
Adenoidectomy

Refer to **DRG 057.**

MDC 03	RW$ 0.2643	Surgical	Outlier Cutoff 3	Mean LOS 1.5

Tonsillectomy and/or Adenoidectomy – Age 0–17

Refer to **DRG 057.**

DETAILS TO CONSIDER

The reader is referred to pediatric texts for additional information.

DRG 061

MDC 03	RW$ 0.4273	Surgical	Outlier Cutoff 9	Mean LOS 2.1

Myringotomy – Age > = 18

OPERATIVE PROCEDURES WITH POTENTIAL HOME CARE NEEDS

Myringotomy with intubation

DETAILS TO CONSIDER

This is a relatively rare adult procedure.

POTENTIAL HOME CARE PROBLEM

Health management deficit.

PLAN

Assess understanding of need for medical follow-up. Teach signs and symptoms requiring follow-up including: vertigo, headache, vomiting, slow pulse rate.

DRG 062

MDC 03	RW$ 0.3121	Surgical	Outlier Cutoff 3	Mean LOS 1.3

Myringotomy – Age 0–17

Same as **DRG 062.**

DETAILS TO CONSIDER

The reader is referred to pediatric texts for additional information.

MDC 03	RW$ 1.1090	Surgical	Outlier Cutoff 26	Mean LOS 5.8

Other Ear, Nose and Throat Operating Room Procedures

OPERATIVE PROCEDURES WITH POTENTIAL HOME CARE NEEDS

Acoustic neuroma
Uvula procedures
Epistaxis control
Gingioplasty
Open reduction of facial bone fracture
Esophageal web incision

DETAILS TO CONSIDER

The procedures in this DRG vary in need for follow-up care. The long-term needs depend on the underlying disease. Most procedures are done for an acute condition.

In acoustic neuroma the patient may be rendered deaf on the affected side.

MDC 03	RW$ 1.0812	Medical	Outlier Cutoff 26	Mean LOS 5.7

Ear, Nose and Throat Malignancy

DIAGNOSES WITH POTENTIAL HOME CARE NEEDS

Cancer of the: tongue; nasopharynx; oral/pharynx; head, face, neck

See **DRG 049.**

DETAILS TO CONSIDER

The long-term needs of these patients depend on the site of the lesion, whether it is a primary or metastatic lesion and the choice of therapy.

DRG 065

MDC 03   **RW$ 0.4857**   **Medical**   **Outlier Cutoff 17**   **Mean LOS 4.6**

Dysequilibrium

DIAGNOSES WITH POTENTIAL HOME CARE NEEDS

Meniere's disease
Labyrinthitis
Dizziness and giddiness

DETAILS TO CONSIDER

Conditions in this group may be chronic, and the treatment may be only minimally effective. Long-term goals include preventing injury to the patient or others during a period of dizziness.

POTENTIAL HOME CARE PROBLEMS	PLAN
1. Health management deficit secondary to attempting to prevent acute attacks.	Control environmental factors causing stress or fatigue. Assess safety related to vertigo and dizziness. Slow body movements to avoid precipitation of attack. Stop smoking.
2. Alteration in nutrition.	Eliminate stimulants, i.e. coffee, tea and chocolate.
3. Pain management.	Take medications as ordered. The patient may use diuretics to avoid fullness in the ear.

DRG 066

MDC 03   **RW$ 0.4116**   **Medical**   **Outlier Cutoff 15**   **Mean LOS 3.7**

Epistaxis

DIAGNOSIS WITH POTENTIAL HOME CARE NEEDS

Epistaxis

DETAILS TO CONSIDER

Epistaxis severe enough to result in hospital admission can be associated with underlying disease.

POTENTIAL HOME CARE PROBLEM	PLAN
Health management deficit.	Emphasize importance of ongoing outpatient care, especially if epistaxis is caused by an underlying systemic disease. Instruct patient to try to prevent head colds and nose trauma. Avoid activity that increases pressure in the nose. Soften crust around nose with vaseline. Promote good mouth care.

MDC 03   **RW$ 0.6762**   **Medical**   **Outlier Cutoff 17**   **Mean LOS 4.3**

Epiglottitis

DIAGNOSES WITH POTENTIAL HOME CARE NEEDS

Epiglottitis with obstruction
Epiglottitis without obstruction

DETAILS TO CONSIDER

This is a relatively rare, although serious, condition, usually of the preschool child. The reader is referred to pediatric texts for additional information.

MDC 03   **RW$ 0.6289**   **Medical**   **Outlier Cutoff 22**   **Mean LOS 6.0**

Otitis Media and Upper Respiratory Infection
Age $>$ = 70 and/or CC

DIAGNOSES WITH POTENTIAL HOME CARE NEEDS

Otitis media
Upper respiratory infection

DETAILS TO CONSIDER

The long-term needs of the patient in this group will depend on the complication and/or comorbidity. These conditions are usually acute and of short duration; thus they should not have long-term effects.

MDC 03   **RW$ 0.5417**   **Medical**   **Outlier Cutoff 19**   **Mean LOS 4.8**

Otitis Media and Upper Respiratory Infection
Age 18–69 w/o CC

Refer to **DRG 068**.

DRG 070

MDC 03	RW$ 0.3697	Medical	Outlier Cutoff 10	Mean LOS 3.1

Otitis Media and Upper Respiratory Infection – Age 0–17

Refer to **DRG 068**.

DETAILS TO CONSIDER

The reader is referred to pediatric texts for additional information.

DRG 071

MDC 03	RW$ 0.3589	Medical	Outlier Cutoff 9	Mean LOS 2.9

Laryngotracheitis

DIAGNOSES WITH POTENTIAL HOME CARE NEEDS

Laryngotracheitis with obstruction.
Laryngotracheitis without obstruction

DETAILS TO CONSIDER

Usually patients with this diagnosis are young children. The reader is referred to pediatric texts for additional information.

DRG 072

MDC 03	RW$ 0.4857	Medical	Outlier Cutoff 18	Mean LOS 3.8

Nasal Trauma and Deformity

DIAGNOSES WITH POTENTIAL HOME CARE NEEDS

Deviated nasal septum
Nasal fracture — closed and open
Foreign body in nose

DETAILS TO CONSIDER

The patient with nasal trauma must be observed for signs and symptoms of concussion and for trauma of the brain and tissues posterior to the nose. Follow-up care will depend on the severity of the injury.

MDC 03	RW$ 0.5217	Medical	Outlier Cutoff 17	Mean LOS 3.5

Other Ear, Nose and Throat Diagnoses – Age > = 18

DIAGNOSES WITH POTENTIAL HOME CARE NEEDS

TB of organ
Hearing loss
Anomalies of ear bones

DETAILS TO CONSIDER

Long-term needs will depend on underlying cause of condition and whether both ears are affected.

MDC 03	RW$ 0.3463	Medical	Outlier Cutoff 9	Mean LOS 2.1

Other Ear, Nose and Throat Diagnoses – Age 0–17

Same as **DRG 073**.

DETAILS TO CONSIDER

The reader is referred to pediatric texts for further information.

4 MDC 04
DISEASES AND DISORDERS OF THE RESPIRATORY SYSTEM

SURGICAL GROUPINGS (3 DRGs)

Major Chest Procedures

OR Procedures on the Respiratory System

MEDICAL GROUPINGS (25 DRGs)

Pulmonary Embolism

Respiratory Infections and Inflammations

Respiratory Neoplasms

Major Chest Trauma

Pleural Effusion

Pulmonary Edema and Respiratory Failure

Chronic Obstructive Pulmonary Disease

Simple Pneumonia and Pleurisy

Interstitial Lung Disease

Pneumothorax

Bronchitis and Asthma

Respiratory Signs and Symptoms

MASTER HOME CARE PLANNING GUIDE
FOR CONDITIONS OF THE RESPIRATORY SYSTEM

	Pattern	Assessment Factors	Plan
1.	Health management deficit	Is the disease chronic or acute? What has been the course of the disease, and what is the prognosis? Has the patient become debilitated, unable to care for self or others? Is the patient's living/working environment conducive to recovery? If not, can effective change be instituted? Has patient's employment been affected by disease? Is patient/caregiver able to comply with medical regime?	Interview patient and family. Review health care regime with patient/caregiver. Make referrals to home care agency, social services, etc., if indicated.
2.	Infection	Does patient's disease make him/her more susceptible to infection? What are the implications of infection in this compromised respiratory state? Is patient an infectious risk to others?	See specific DRG.
3.	Physical injury	Is patient's disease apt to place him/her at risk of suffocation or sudden and severe respiratory distress?	May need medical alert bracelet; instruction in regard to importance of practicing safety measures to maintain patent airway. See specific DRG.
4.	Potential fluid volume deficit	Adequate hydration is important in order to facilitate secretion removal. Must also consider fluid overload as pulmonary and cardiac systems are interdependent.	See specific DRG.
5.	Alteration in nutrition	Assess patient's nutritional status. Obesity is detrimental to optimum air exchange. Nutritional deficit is common in chronic respiratory disease states. Acute illness/surgery may also demand increased caloric protein, CHO consumption to heal wounds. Fatigue and/or SOB may make meal preparation and eating itself difficult.	Assess patient's nutritional status and ability to obtain and prepare meals. Provide dietary instructions and assistance in the home where indicated. See specific DRG.
6.	Alteration in skin integrity	Is the patient being discharged with an open wound? Assess ability to care for wound and knowledge of symptoms to report to physician.	See specific DRG.
7.	Alteration in elimination	Altered nutritional status and decreased activity create potential for constipation.	Determine patient's normal bowel pattern. Review with patient/caregiver effects of analgesics, decreased activity, poor dietary habits or bowel elimination. Provide instructions regarding measures to counteract constipation.

8. Activity — exercise	Achievement of maximum level of physical activity is important to physical recovery and mental well-being. Time must be planned carefully to conserve energy.	Assist patient/family in planning alternating schedule of rest and activity. Stress importance of setting realistic attainable goals.
9. Potential for ineffective clearance	Maintenance of patent airway and removal of secretions is vital in order to maximize efficiency of an already compromised respiratory system and prevent extension of disease.	See specific DRG.
10. Alteration in breathing pattern	Patient may have developed compensatory breathing pattern. Need to be instructed in most efficient use of accessory muscles, coughing and breathing techniques to conserve energy. Alteration in breathing pattern may herald onset of respiratory distress.	Assess patient's usual breathing pattern and patient's knowledge of symptoms to report to physician. Instruct in breathing exercises if indicated.
11. Home maintenance management deficit	Chronic respiratory illness may have catastrophic effect on patient's ability to care for self/family.	Interview patient/family to determine living arrangements, bathroom facilities, ability to obtain and prepare meals, transportation for follow-up medical care. In determining home care needs, consider: • level of care needed. • assistive devices needed to cope with ADL. • availability of caregiver/significant others. • need for homemaker services.
12. Pain management	Assess patient's level of pain. Pain may cause patient to splint chest, thereby decreasing pulmonary expansion. Pain may also herald the onset of acute respiratory distress.	Discuss use of analgesics with patient. Instruct patient regarding signs to report to physician. See specific DRG.
13. Knowledge deficit	Outlook for chronic respiratory disease is dependent on scrupulous attention to health care regime. Respiratory setbacks may be irreversible. Prevention is vital.	Assess patient/caregiver level of knowledge regarding planned health care regime. Provide instruction and obtain feedback.
14. Sleep pattern disturbance	Paroxysmal Nocturnal Dyspnea (PND), orthopnea, and increased secretions may interfere with patient's sleep.	See specific DRG.
15. Anxiety	Anxiety may precipitate respiratory symptoms. Need to increase patient's ability to cope with stress.	See specific DRG.

16. Depression	Depression is common in chronic respiratory disease. Loss of health and independence, repeated hospitalizations and exacerbation of symptoms all contribute to depression. Patient with newly diagnosed respiratory illness may also be depressed.	Assess availability of patient support systems. Encourage maximum activity level (within patient's tolerance) to combat depression. Determine need for follow-up mental health care.
17. Coping tolerance	Extent, duration and prognosis of disease may affect patient's ability to care for self/others.	Assess patient/family's ability to cope with illness. Consider financial, home, work, social, medical implications of diagnosis. Make appropriate referrals (community agencies, counseling, etc.).

DRG 075

MDC 04	RW$ 2.6044	Surgical	Outlier Cutoff 34	Mean LOS 14.4

Major Chest Procedures

OPERATIVE PROCEDURES WITH POTENTIAL HOME CARE NEEDS

Thymectomy
Pneumonectomy
Lobectomy or segmental lung resection
Decortication of the lung
Diaphragmatic pacemaker

DETAILS TO CONSIDER

Long-term needs depend on underlying pathology, extent of preexisting pulmonary compromise and postoperative pulmonary function.

POTENTIAL HOME CARE PROBLEMS

PLAN

1. Health management deficit.

Assess patient's understanding of effect of decreased pulmonary capacity. Instruct patient to avoid smoking and smoke pollution (smoking decreases airflow to lungs and paralyzes cilia). Avoid air pollution, i.e. smog, heavy traffic, aerosol sprays, chemical fumes, persons with URIs. Discuss with patient and/or caregiver need for medical follow-up, treatments, radiation, etc.

2. Nutritional deficit.

Determine patient's usual dietary pattern. Assess need for dietary instruction to increase protein and caloric consumption to promote wound healing and combat infection.

2a. Fluid volume.

Stress importance of adequate fluid intake to maintain fluid balance to facilitate secretion removal.

3. Alteration in bowel elimination pattern: potential for constipation.

Interview patient to determine normal bowel pattern. Stress effect of surgery, analgesics, decreased activity in contributing to constipation. Instruct patient to increase dietary fiber, bulk, use analgesics only as needed, increase activity to level of tolerance. Instruct patient in conservative use of laxatives (avoid mineral oil as it interferes with the absorption of vitamins A & D).

4. Activity/exercise pattern: potential for decreased tolerance.

Interview patient to assess premorbid level of activity. Instruct patient to increase activity to tolerance level (onset of fatigue, SOB, etc.). Encourage patient and caregiver to stagger activities with periods of rest and to set attainable goals to encourage increasing exercise and coping with activities of daily life.

5. Ineffective airway clearance.

Instruct patient to note and report to physician unusual amount and/or character of secretions (i.e. purulent, bloody, frothy, tenacious, etc.), difficulty raising secretions or clearing airway. Adequate humidity should be maintained in the home to facilitate raising secretions.

6. Ineffective breathing pattern.

Instruct patient to note and report to physician any unusual SOB, wheeze, cough, cyanosis and temperature (note causative factors, duration and severity of symptom). Encourage maximum activity level and frequent change of position to promote optimum lung expansion. Advise patient/caregiver to be aware of changes in patient's normal breathing pattern (use of accessory muscles, abdominal breathing, visible signs of respiratory distress, SOB, etc.).

7. Home care management deficit.

Interview patient/family to determine living arrangements and environment. Consider:
- diagnosis and prognosis.
- level of care needs.
- ability and availability of caregiver and community agencies.

8. Pain control.

Instruct patient to distinguish between normal postoperative pain and onset of unusual pain. Instruct patient to describe pain (e.g. sharp, dull, worse on inspiration, relieved with change in position, etc.) and notify physician. Discuss with patient and/or caregiver use of analgesics — include schedule and side effects.

9. Sleep-rest pattern.

Determine according to surgery and diagnoses if lying on either side is preferable to promote lung expansion and/or drainage. Elevating the head of the bed may be more comfortable in some cases.

10. Self-esteem disturbance.

Decreased tolerance for work or activities of daily life may be disturbing. Assist patient/family in setting realistic and attainable goals to promote feelings of self-worth.

REFERRAL INFORMATION

Refer to home care agency if patient has need for follow-up care. This will depend on the patient's health history, diagnosis and prognosis, family situation and living arrangements. Also assess the need for durable medical equipment such as an electric bed, oxygen equipment or assistive devices for ambulation or bathing.

DRG 076

MDC 04   **RW$ 1.8734**   **Surgical**   **Outlier Cutoff 31**   **Mean LOS 10.6**

Operating Room Procedures on the Respiratory System Except Major Chest with CC

OPERATIVE PROCEDURES WITH POTENTIAL HOME CARE NEEDS

Laryngectomy
Lymph node biopsy
Chest cage procedures
Permanent tracheostomy

DETAILS TO CONSIDER

Patient with comorbidity or complication. Long-term needs depend on underlying disease, prognosis, age, and ability of the patient to comply with medical regime. Tracheostomy/laryngectomy may be associated with a history of alcohol/tobacco abuse; possibility of metastatic disease exists.

POTENTIAL HOME CARE PROBLEMS

1. Health management deficit.

1a. Potential for physical injury.
Potential for suffocation.

2. Nutrition deficit.

2a. Fluid volume.

PLAN

Assess patient's understanding of care of laryngectomy/tracheotomy and follow-up medical care (radiation, chemotherapy medication). Instruct patient to avoid smoking and smoke pollution. Avoid air pollution, smog, aerosol sprays, chemical fumes, persons with upper respiratory infections.

Patient to wear medical alert bracelet. Instruct patient/family regarding safety measures for tracheotomy — need for patent airway at all times, potential for tissue trauma from suctioning, absence of filtering and humidifying function of nose, need to avoid water into stoma (no swimming, careful showers, electric razor only around stoma for men).

Assess patient's premorbid dietary pattern. Develop with patient/caregiver dietary plan to meet increased protein and caloric requirement toward healing. Loss of sense of smell may decrease appetite. Stress importance of eating. Assess patient/caregiver ability to administer tube feedings, if ordered. Patient/caregiver should be able to perform site care if gastrostomy tube is present; should be able to demonstrate principles of safe administration of tube feedings.

Stress importance of adequate hydration in facilitating secretion removal. Instruct patient to maintain proper body alignment while eating to decrease the risk of aspiration. Swallowing thin liquids may be more difficult than semi-solids (custard, ice cream, gelatin).

3. Alteration in bowel elimination: potential for constipation/diarrhea.	Patient may experience alteration in bowel habits and changes in dietary pattern. Instruct patient in diet adequate to resolve condition. Provide information on dietary supplements relating to constipation/diarrhea. (Dehydration is of special significance to patient — have patient report to physician diarrhea that does not respond to treatment.)
4. Ineffective airway clearance.	Instruct patient/caregiver in suctioning technique. Assess ability to perform procedure. Determine need for home care equipment (suction apparatus, catheters, dressings, tapes, vaporizers, oxygen). Instruct patient to note amount and character of secretions, presence of bleeding and to report any change in above to physician.
5. Pain control.	Decreased chest movement accompanied by decreased lung expansion may predispose patient to atelectasis/pneumonia. Instruct patient to maintain adequate pain control with minimum effective medication. Assess patient/family understanding of use of analgesics. Encourage exercise to promote increased tidal volume.
6. Alteration in body image.	Encourage patient/family to verbalize feelings. Assess usefulness of contact with patient with similar surgery. Encourage rapid return to normal ADL. Provide information regarding acceptable tracheostomy coverings (e.g. scarves, decorative dressings, etc.).
7. Grieving.	Assist patient/family through grieving process. Assess need for follow-up mental health care.
8. Social isolation related to impaired verbal communication.	Encourage reintegration of patient into social environment to decrease effect of impaired communication. Assess need for instruction in alternate methods of speech (esophageal, mechanical devices).

REFERRAL INFORMATION

Secure pertinent health history and prognosis, pertinent family situation and living arrangements, current hospitalization history — course of illness, patient/caregiver level of ability regarding care of tracheotomy feedings; durable medical equipment if needed — humidifier, suction equipment, tracheotomy supplies, supplemental feedings, dressing supplies, assistive devices for ADL.

DRG 077

MDC 04	RW$ 1.8178	Surgical	Outlier Cutoff 30	Mean LOS 9.5

Operating Procedures on Respiratory System Except Major Chest w/o CC

OPERATIVE PROCEDURES WITH POTENTIAL HOME CARE NEEDS

Same as **DRG 076.**

DETAILS TO CONSIDER

Patient without comorbidity or complications.

See **DRG 076.**

DRG 078

MDC 04	RW$ 1.4095	Medical	Outlier Cutoff 30	Mean LOS 10.4

Pulmonary Embolism

PRINCIPAL DIAGNOSES WITH POTENTIAL HOME CARE NEEDS

Pulmonary embolism/infarction
Air embolism
Fat embolism

DETAILS TO CONSIDER

Long-term needs depend on presence of related disease states (CHF, venostases) prognosis and likelihood of recurrence.

POTENTIAL HOME CARE PROBLEMS / PLAN

POTENTIAL HOME CARE PROBLEMS	PLAN
1. Health management deficit related to need for long-term preventive measures.	Assess contributing factors relating to diagnoses (e.g. pulmonary embolus may be related to atrial fibrillation with CHF, stasis of peripheral vascular bed, air embolus secondary to diving). Assess patient's understanding of causative factors and ability to comply with medical regime to decrease risk of recurrence.
2. Alteration in nutrition — obesity.	Determine if there is a need for weight reduction, dietary instruction. (Obesity is a contributing factor in development of PE)

3. Activity/exercise pattern.

Interview patient: define patterns of activity/exercises that contribute to disease. Develop alternate methods of activity to decrease risk of reembolization (e.g. elevate legs 15° when recumbent, avoid prolonged sitting, standing).

4. Knowledge deficit related to anticoagulant therapy; antiembolism measures.

Assess patient's understanding of therapy and ability to comply with follow-up lab studies. Consider:
- varied dosage and scheduling of medication.
- necessity for patient levels (and ability of patient to get to lab).
- precautions to be followed while on anticoagulants (no ASA or over-the-counter drugs containing ASA, electric razor for men, need to avoid sharp tools, contact sports, etc.).
- avoidance of excessive Vitamin K in diet.
- need to inform physician prior to taking any other medication.
- need to report to physician bruises, bleeding from mucous membranes, bloody urine or bowel movements, nosebleeds, etc.

Instruct patient in proper use of antiembolism stockings, if ordered.

5. Potential for impaired thought process.

Possible mental confusion following development of fat embolus. Ensure that family/caregiver will be available to patient. Provide for patient safety at home.

DRG 079

MDC 04   **RW$ 1.7982**   **Medical**   **Outlier Cutoff 31**   **Mean LOS 11.2**

Respiratory Infections and Inflammations – Age > = 70 and/or CC

PRINCIPAL DIAGNOSES WITH POTENTIAL HOME CARE NEEDS

Tuberculosis
Pneumonia
Abscess of Lune
Mediastinitis

DETAILS TO CONSIDER

Patient is 70 or older with comorbidity and/or complications. Long-term needs depend on extent of disease and prognosis (mediastinitis may be chronic or acute).

POTENTIAL HOME CARE PROBLEMS	PLAN
1. Health management deficit secondary to age of patient and presence of other illness.	Assess patient's ability to follow health regime and cope with ADL (see **DRG 075**). Assess availability of support systems. Instruct patient and caregiver regarding medications.
2. Potential for infection.	Determine need to report contacts of patient who has documented tuberculosis. Instruct patient/family to dispose of secretions properly: • use disposable tissues. • use tissue once. • dispose of in paper bag. • cover mouth and nose when coughing. • wash hands after handling secretions. • continue medications as ordered. • avoid persons with URIs.
3. Potential for: Nutritional deficit.	Instruct patient in high carbohydrate diet. Encourage good oral hygiene prior to meals if shortness of breath is a problem while eating.
3a. Fluid volume deficit.	Adequate hydration is important to facilitate removal of secretions. Instruct patient to force fluids unless constipated.
4. Activity/exercise potential for decreased tolerance.	Depending on extent and duration of disease, adequate oxygenation may be a problem. Assist patient/caregiver in planning periods of rest between activities. Increase level of activity gradually.
5. Potential for ineffective airway clearance.	Stress importance of home environment — adequate humidity, decreased air pollution. Assess patient's ability to perform effective postural drainage, cough and deep breathing techniques. Encourage activity and change in position to promote drainage. Instruct patient to report unusual secretions to physician (note color, amount, character, presence of blood).

| MDC 04 | RW$ 1.7445 | Medical | Outlier Cutoff 31 | Mean LOS 10.9 |

Respiratory Infections and Inflammations – Age 18–69 w/o CC

See **DRG 079.**

| MDC 04 | RW$ 0.8743 | Medical | Outlier Cutoff 26 | Mean LOS 6.1 |

Respiratory Infections and Inflammations – Age 0–17

PRINCIPAL DIAGNOSIS WITH POTENTIAL HOME CARE NEEDS
See **DRG 079.**

DETAILS TO CONSIDER

Patient is under 18. Education of parent/caregiver is important to ensure compliance with health care regimen. Special consideration of fluid balance, medication dosage, notation of exacerbation of symptoms, positioning, postural drainage, and breathing exercises should be taken.

See **DRG 079** and **DRG 091.**

DRG 082

Respiratory Neoplasms

PRINCIPAL DIAGNOSES WITH POTENTIAL HOME CARE NEEDS

Malignant neoplasms: trachea, bronchus, lung pleura, mediastinum, thorax
Secondary neoplasms

DETAILS TO CONSIDER

Long-term needs are dependent on diagnosis, prognosis, site and extent of disease, plan of health care follow-up, and ability of the patient to comply with care. Site of primary disease must also be considered in relation to metastatic lesions (see appropriate DRGs). Pleural neoplasms may represent as pleural effusion (see **DRG 085**).

POTENTIAL HOME CARE PROBLEMS

PLAN

1. Health management deficit.

Assess patient's understanding of need for follow-up health care (radiation, chemotherapy). Assess patient/family ability to obtain and comply with care. Consider transportation and community service. Assess patient's ability to care for self and availability of significant others.

2. Alteration in nutrition: Potential for deficit.

Patient often seeks treatment for respiratory neoplasms when weight loss and anorexia are already established. Do baseline nutritional assessment. Provide dietary instruction. Encourage high protein, high caloric meals and vitamin supplements indicated. If SOB is a problem, encourage small, frequent meals. Determine ability of patient to obtain and/or prepare meals. Make referral if indicated for assistance.

2a. Potential for fluid volume deficit.

Encourage adequate fluids unless contraindicated to facilitate removal of secretions.

3. Potential for ineffective airway clearance.

Stress need for adequate humidity, fluids, medications (if ordered) to facilitate secretion removal. Instruct patient to notify physician of change in amount and/or character of secretions. Determine need for suction equipment.

3a. Potential for ineffective breathing pattern.

Assess patient's usual breathing pattern. Anticipate problems with decreased aeration with growing tumor. Instruct patient to notify physician of increase in SOB, DOE, amount and/or character of secretions, presence of blood in secretion, development of wheeze and/or labored respirations. Determine need for oxygen equipment. Encourage effective C&DB exercises, postural drainage. Instruct family/caregiver if indicated.

4. Pain management.

Assess patient's understanding of use of analgesics. Encourage minimum effective dose as overuse may decrease respiratory drive.

5. Anxiety.

Determine level of anxiety. Provide information regarding treatment plan to decrease anxiety. Determine need for further treatment of anxiety through use of medication and/or therapy.

6. Grief.

Patient/family may experience grief over loss of health, especially if disease represents metastasis of primary lesion. Assess where patient/family is in the grieving process. Determine need for ongoing therapy.

REFERRAL INFORMATION

Background information — pertinent health history, diagnoses and prognosis; pertinent family situation and availability of significant others. Current hospitalization history including complications and follow-up medical care. Durable medical eqipment if indicated — oxygen equipment, suction equipment, assistive devices needed for ADL. Referrals to community agencies — Meals-on-Wheels; transportation services for follow-up radiation, medical care.

DRG 083

MDC 04	RW$ 0.9809	Medical	Outlier Cutoff 28	Mean LOS 8.1

Major Chest Trauma – Age > = 70 and/or CC

PRINCIPAL DIAGNOSES WITH POTENTIAL HOME CARE NEEDS

Fractured multiple ribs
Flail chest
Lung laceration
Diaphragm injury
Open wound of trachea

DETAILS TO CONSIDER

Patient is 70 or older with comorbidity or complications. Of special concern is patient with preexisting pulmonary or cardiac disease as chest trauma is further insult to compromised respiratory function.

POTENTIAL HOME CARE PROBLEMS

PLAN

1. Health management deficit secondary to age of patient or other illness.

Assess patient's ability to comply with health regime for other illness and impact of present illness on ability to care for self.

2. Potential for physical injury.

Advise patient to avoid risk of further injury. Instruct to notify physician immediately if symptoms of pneumothorax develop.

3.	Alteration in bowel elimination: potential for constipation secondary to analgesic use.	Encourage adequate fluid and bulk in diet. Instruct patient as to the minimum effective dose of pain medication and gradually increase activity level. Over the counter laxatives may be needed unless contraindicated.
4.	Potential for ineffective airway clearance.	Injuries to chest inhibit expansion because of pain. Therefore, encourage patient to effectively cough and deep breathe every 2–3 hours. Instruct patient to maintain adequate humidity in environment to facilitate removal of secretions. Teach patient to splint chest while attempting to cough. Instruct patient in proper postural drainage if ordered.
5.	Potential for ineffective breathing pattern.	Encourage patient to change position frequently and increase tolerance of activity to promote maximum lung expansion.
6.	Pain management.	Unstable rib movement may cause pain with deep respiration and/or cough. Instruct patient to use analgesics prior to vigorous respiratory exercises. Encourage patient to cough and deep breathe frequently. Reassure patient the pain will progressively improve.

DRG 084

MDC 04	RW$ 0.7738	Medical	Outlier Cutoff 22	Mean LOS 5.3

Major Chest Trauma – Age < 70 w/o CC

PRINCIPAL DIAGNOSIS WITH POTENTIAL HOME CARE NEEDS

See **DRG 083.**

DETAILS TO CONSIDER

Stress importance of avoiding possibility of further injury through bodily contact, sports participation, etc., especially in younger patients.

Pleural Effusion – Age > = 70 and/or CC

PRINCIPAL DIAGNOSIS WITH POTENTIAL HOME CARE NEEDS

Pleural effusion

See **DRG 084.**

DETAILS TO CONSIDER

Patient is 70 or older with comorbidity or complications. Consider primary disease. Except for pleural neoplasms, pleural effusion is always secondary to a disease process outside the pleura — lung, mediastinum, subdiaphragmatic space, or esophagus. Pneumonia or tuberculosis may be present (see specific DRG).

POTENTIAL HOME CARE PROBLEMS	PLAN
1. Health management deficit secondary to patient age and other illness.	Assess patient's level of understanding of follow-up health care. Assess impact of disease on patient's ability to care for self and/or others.
2. Potential for alteration in fluid balance.	If noninflammatory pleural effusion is present, it may be associated with sodium retention. Patient may present generalized edema. Do patient assessment and instruct in fluid restriction if prescribed. Have patient keep record of daily weights and report weight gain to physician.
3. Potential for alteration in nutrition.	Instruct in low sodium diet, if indicated.
4. Alteration in breathing pattern.	Depending on amount of fluid in pleural space, slowly evolving effusion may be tolerated by patient. A large amount of exudate, however, may precipitate respiratory distress. Instruct patient to note and report to physician symptoms of recurring effusion (localized chest pain, dyspnea, cough, fatigue, asymmetrical expansion of chest).
5. Pain management.	Patient may experience chest pain if effusion is preceded by a dry pleurisy. Instruct patient to splint chest with coughing and deep breathing exercises. Assess patient's level of understanding of analgesics.
6. Potential for sleep/rest disturbance.	Pleural fluid collects in dependent position. Head of bed may need to be elevated. Assess and advise patient of best position for rest and maximum lung expansion.

REFERRAL INFORMATION

No referral needed unless patient was receiving home care services for preexisting disease, or unless fatigue, weakness interfere with patient's ability to care for self.

DRG 086

MDC 04   **RW$ 1.1217**   **Medical**   **Outlier Cutoff 28**   **Mean LOS 7.6**

Pleural Effusion – Age < 70 w/o CC

See **DRG 085.**

DRG 087

MDC 04   **RW$ 1.5529**   **Medical**   **Outlier Cutoff 28**   **Mean LOS 7.7**

Pulmonary Edema and Respiratory Failure

PRINCIPAL DIAGNOSIS WITH POTENTIAL HOME CARE NEEDS

Pulmonary edema and respiratory failure

DETAILS TO CONSIDER

Long-term health care needs will be affected by presence of accompanying cardiac disease (see appropriate DRG). Do complete cardiac respiratory assessment before determining long-term needs. Good patient/caregiver education is of special importance in preventing exacerbations of symptoms in chronic respiratory failure.

POTENTIAL HOME CARE PROBLEMS	PLAN
1. Health management deficit related to need for long-term follow-up.	Assess patient/caregiver understanding of health care regime. Note instructions to maintain healthy environment — avoid persons with URI (even a common cold may cause permanent lung damage), avoid air pollution, smoking, respiratory irritants.
2. Potential for alteration in fluid balance.	Adequate hydration is important to facilitate secretion removal. Avoidance of fluid overload is also important to prevent pulmonary congestion. Determine fluid needs and instruct patient/caregiver.
3. Potential for alteration in nutrition.	Instruct patient in sodium restricted diet if indicated.
4. Potential for decreased activity tolerance.	Increasing activity/independence to tolerance is vital. Oxygen may be needed temporarily at home. Instruct patient to stagger rest and work periods.
4a. Potential for self-care deficit.	Assess level of needs. May require assistive devices to maintain independence in ADL.

5. Potential for ineffective airway clearance.	Determine need for assistive respiratory equipment (i.e. oxygen, IPPB equipment). Instruct patient in effective coughing and breathing techniques. Assess patient's ability to note and report changes in health status (changes in secretions, breathing pattern, level of activity tolerance). Instruct patient to report purulent secretions to physician immediately. Early treatment of infection is important.
6. Potential for ineffective breathing pattern.	Assess patient's ability to perform breathing exercises to increase lung expansion, decrease work of accessory muscles, and improve functioning of diaphragm.
7. Knowledge deficit secondary to complex health care needs.	Interview patient and review record to determine medication regimen. Instruct patient in medication usage, side effects, expected outcome. Include diuretics, cardiac medications, electrolyte supplements, as well as pulmonary medications if ordered. Instruct patient to check weight and report increase to physician. Assess patient's ability to effectively use respiratory equipment provided.
8. Sleep/rest pattern disturbance secondary to PND.	Instruct patient to maintain fluid balance. Use bronchodilators if ordered, elevate head of bed, maintain healthy environment.

REFERRAL INFORMATION

Home care nursing, respiratory therapist, physiotherapist. Background information-pertinent health history and prognosis, pertinent living and environmental considerations — include ability of patient to care for self. Current hospitalization history including complications, course of illness, patient's level of ability to cope with ADL. Durable medical equipment: assistive devices for self-care, oxygen equipment (including IPPB, aerosol equipment).

DRG 088

Chronic Obstructive Pulmonary Disease

PRINCIPAL DIAGNOSES WITH POTENTIAL HOME CARE NEEDS

Emphysema
Bronchiectasis

DETAILS TO CONSIDER

Both emphysema and bronchiectasis are chronic diseases. Patient education to prevent exacerbations of symptoms is of paramount importance. Duration and extent of disease will affect long-term needs.

POTENTIAL HOME CARE PROBLEMS	PLAN
1. Health management deficit.	Assess patient's understanding of need for follow-up care and impact of disease on ability to care for and support self (see **DRG 075** Health Mgt. Deficit).
2. Potential for infection to self and others.	Instruct patient to avoid persons with URIs. Important to report first symptoms of URI to physician immediately (fever, sore throat, increased dyspnea, sinusitis). Instruct patient to dispose of secretions properly (see **DRG 079**).
3. Potential for fluid volume deficit.	Adequate hydration important to facilitate removal of secretions. Instruct patient to force fluids unless contraindicated.
4. Potential for nutritional deficit secondary to weight loss caused by increased energy expenditure from increased work of breathing; also decreased caloric consumption secondary to air swallowing, SOB while eating, nausea.	Instruct in high protein, high caloric diet as ordered. Encourage good oral hygiene prior to meals. Instruct patient to rest before meals if SOB is a problem while eating. Assess patient's ability to obtain and/or prepare meals. Arrange for assistance if indicated.
5. Potential for alteration in bowel elimination: constipation as a result of inactivity and altered status.	Instruct patient in diet with adequate bulk and fluids. Over-the-counter laxatives may be needed. Caution patient regarding abuse.
6. Potential for decreased activity tolerance.	Increasing patient's activity to tolerance level is important. Assist patient/family in planning rest periods alternating with activities. Interview patient/family and assist in planning ADL to conserve patient's energy and maximize independence.
7. Potential for ineffective airway clearance.	Assess patient's understanding of and ability to perform effective postural drainage, coughing and deep breathing.

8. Potential for ineffective breathing pattern.

Breathing exercises and coughing techniques to avoid further air-trapping are important. Assess patient's ability to comply with prescribed breathing exercise program. Instruct patient to avoid factors which will increase the work of breathing (i.e. cold air, increased air pollution index).

9. Potential for self-care deficit related to fatigue, SOB, muscle waste (as result of poor nutrition).

Assess need for assistive devices to conserve patient's energy and maximize independence.

10. Knowledge deficit relating to need for long-term follow-up medical care.

Assess patient/caregiver understanding of medical regime (special attention to medications, exercise, maintenance of healthy environment, conservation of energy).

11. Depression: related to chronic illness and decreased ability to maintain usual level of activity/independence.

Depression common. Assess need for follow-up therapy. Instruct caregiver/family in importance of assisting patient to achieve and maintain maximum level of activity (within patient's tolerance) in order to combat depression.

12. Coping tolerance — secondary to chronic illness with implications for effect on family finances, activities, etc.

Interview patient/family. Assess need for social service referral.

REFERRAL INFORMATION

Assess need for referrals to home care nurse, respiratory therapist, social worker, mental health therapist. Background information: pertinent health history and prognosis; pertinent family situation and living arrangements. Current hospitalizaiton: course of illness, including cause of exacerbation of symptoms and medical regimen to be followed. Durable medical equipment: assistive devices, if any for ADL; oxygen equipment, respiratory equipment.

DRG 089

MDC 04   RW$ 1.1029   Medical   Outlier Cutoff 29   Mean LOS 8.5

Simple Pneumonia and Pleurisy – Age ≥ 70 and/or CC

PRINCIPAL DIAGNOSIS WITH POTENTIAL HOME CARE NEEDS

Simple pneumonia and pleurisy

DETAILS TO CONSIDER

Patient is 70 or older with comorbidity and/or complications.

POTENTIAL HOME CARE PROBLEMS	PLAN
1. Health management deficit secondary to age of patient and other illness.	Assess patient's ability to comply with health regime and to care for self.
2. Potential for infection.	Instruct patient to avoid persons with URIs.
3. Potential for fluid volume deficit.	Encourage patient to force fluids to facilitate secretion removal unless contraindicated.
4. Alteration in activity tolerance.	Assess patient's level of activity. Encourage increasing activity to tolerance. Plan alternating periods of rest/activity.
5. Potential for ineffective breathing pattern.	Assess patient's understanding of effective coughing, breathing, postural drainage. Instruct patient/caregiver in proper techniques. Encourage frequent pulmonary toilet to promote maximum lung expansion and remove secretions.
6. Self-care deficit related to fatigue, SOB.	Assess patient's ability to care for self. Determine need for assistive devices or community referrals.
7. Pain management secondary to localized chest pain or inspiration occurring with pleurisy.	Instruct patient to splint chest while coughing. Assess knowledge of correct usage of analgesics.
8. Knowledge deficit.	Instruct patient in proper use of antibiotics if continued at home.

REFERRAL INFORMATION

None — unless patient is already receiving services for other illness, or has decrease in ability to care for self.

| MDC 04 | RW$ 0.9849 | Medical | Outlier Cutoff 28 | Mean LOS 7.6 |

Simple Pneumonia and Pleurisy – Age 18–69 w/o CC

See **DRG 089.**

| MDC 04 | RW$ 0.5131 | Medical | Outlier Cutoff 14 | Mean LOS 4.6 |

Simple Pneumonia and Pleurisy – Age 0–17

PRINCIPAL DIAGNOSIS WITH POTENTIAL HOME CARE NEEDS

Simple pneumonia and pleurisy

DETAILS TO CONSIDER

Patient is under 18. Include parent/caregiver in planning health care regime.

POTENTIAL HOME CARE PROBLEMS	PLAN
1. Health management deficit secondary to age of patient.	Assess patient/caregiver ability to comply with health care regimen and meet patient's needs.
2. Potential for infection.	Patient to avoid persons with URIs.
3. Potential for fluid volume deficit.	See **DRG 089.**
4. Alteration in activity/tolerance.	Patient may be on bedrest or decreased activity to combat fatigue and weakness. Assist parent in planning periods of rest to alternate with activity. Interview caregiver to determine if patient's school needs will be met.
5. Potential for ineffective breathing pattern.	See **DRG 089.**
6. Knowledge deficit.	Assess patient/caregiver ability to comply with medication schedule. Antibiotics and aspirin may be prescribed to combat infection and fever. Instruct in proper use, side effects.

DRG 092

MDC 04   **RW$ 1.0370**   **Medical**   **Outlier Cutoff 28**   **Mean LOS 7.8**

Interstitial Lung Disease – Age > = 70 and/or CC

PRINCIPAL DIAGNOSES WITH POTENTIAL HOME CARE NEEDS

Pneumoconiosis
Rheumatoid lung
Systemic sclerosis lung disease

DETAILS TO CONSIDER

Patient is 70 or older with comorbidity and/or complications. Interstitial lung disease may be related to working/living environment. Patient age may make a change in environment difficult.

POTENTIAL HOME CARE PROBLEMS	PLAN
1. Health management deficit secondary to age of patient, other illness, and ability to alter environment.	Assess patient's ability to comply with health regime — and impact of compromised pulmonary function on ability to care for self.
2. Potential for decreased activity tolerance.	Assess patient's level of activity. Encourage periods of rest between activities. Assess patient's ability to cope with ADL — can patient climb stairs, ambulate unassisted, etc.? Determine need for assistive devices.
3. Potential for ineffective breathing pattern — dyspnea due to increasing work of respiratory muscles necessary to move fibrotic lung.	Assess extent of patient's dyspnea. Treatment is symptomatic as disease is irreversible. Encourage patient to practice good pulmonary care (see **DRG 088**).
4. Potential for depression — common as patient's tolerance for activity becomes more limited.	Encourage verbalization. Instruct patient in techniques to improve activity tolerance (see **DRG 088**). Encourage reintegration into family, social, work environment within patient's tolerance. Establish attainable goals with patient. Determine need for mental health follow-up.

| MDC 04 | RW$ 0.9724 | Medical | Outlier Cutoff 27 | Mean LOS 6.9 |

Interstitial Lung Disease – Age < 70 w/o CC

PRINCIPAL DIAGNOSIS WITH POTENTIAL HOME CARE NEEDS

See DRG 092.

DETAILS TO CONSIDER

In this age group, if patient's disease is caused by environmental factors — change in job or home may be needed. Assess impact of such a change on patient/family. Assess financial implications to patient/family and make appropriate referrals if indicated.

| MDC 04 | RW$ 1.4374 | Medical | Outlier Cutoff 29 | Mean LOS 9.2 |

Pneumothorax – Age > = 70 and/or CC

PRINCIPAL DIAGNOSES WITH POTENTIAL HOME CARE NEEDS

Spontaneous pneumothorax
Traumatic pneumothorax/pneumohemothorax

DETAILS TO CONSIDER

Patient is 70 or older with comorbidity and/or complications.

POTENTIAL HOME CARE PROBLEMS	PLAN
1. Health management deficit secondary to age of patient and/or other illness.	Assess patient's ability to follow health regime of preexisting illness and impact of present illness on ability to care for self.
2. Skin integrity impaired.	If patient discharge with open wound — assess patient/caregiver ability to do wound care and understanding of symptoms to report to physician (redness, swelling, drainage, heat, tenderness, fever).
3. Potential for ineffective breathing pattern.	Patient may inhibit chest expansion in order to avoid discomfort. Instruct patient to cough and deep breathe every 2–4 hours to provide maximum lung expansion. Instruct patient in importance of reporting recurrence of respiratory symptoms to physician (sudden localized sharp chest pain, SOB, bloody sputum, fever).
4. Pain management.	Assess patient's understanding of use of analgesics. Instruct patient to use minimum effective dose to promote comfort.

DRG 095

MDC 04	RW$ 1.1252	Medical	Outlier Cutoff 28	Mean LOS 7.7

Pneumothorax – Age < 70 w/o CC

See **DRG 094.**

DRG 096

MDC 04	RW$ 0.7996	Medical	Outlier Cutoff 24	Mean LOS 6.9

Bronchitis and Asthma – Age > = 70 and/or CC

PRINCIPAL DIAGNOSES WITH POTENTIAL HOME CARE NEEDS

Bronchitis
Asthma

DETAILS TO CONSIDER

Patient is 70 or older with comorbidity and/or complications.

POTENTIAL HOME CARE PROBLEMS	PLAN
1. Health management deficit potential related to need for long-term follow-up.	Assess patient's ability to comply with medical regime for other illnesses and impact of present illness on ability to care for self.
2. Potential for infection secondary to decreased capacity of ciliary activity.	Instruct patient to avoid persons with URI and to notify physician at the first sign of URI (fever, sore throat, postnasal drip, increased dyspnea, cough).
3. Potential for increased activity tolerance.	Assess patient's level of activity. Encourage frequent periods of rest. Caution patient to avoid excessive exercise that may precipitate onset/worsening of symptoms.
4. Potential for ineffective airway clearance secondary to production of copious and/or thick sputum.	Instruct patient to maintain adequate humidity in environment. Assess patient understanding and ability to comply with postural drainage, correct coughing and breathing techniques.
5. Potential for alteration in breathing pattern.	Instruct patient to avoid respiratory irritants that may precipitate attack, i.e. allergies, cold temperatures, stress, emotional upset, air/smoke pollution. Assess patient's ability to execute proper breathing/coughing techniques.

6.	Potential for self-care deficit.			Assess patient's ability to care for self in presence of decreased pulmonary capacity and increasing DOE. Assess need for assistive devices.
7.	Knowledge deficit.			Instruct patient in proper use of aerosol medications and/or equipment. Provide information regarding side effects of bronchodilators.
8.	Potential for ineffective stress tolerance.			Assess effectiveness of patient's coping mechanisms as stress/emotional upset may trigger asthma attacks. Assess need for mental health follow-up in dealing with stress.

DRG 097

MDC 04	RW$ 0.7256	Medical	Outlier Cutoff 21	Mean LOS 6.2

Bronchitis and Asthma – Age 18–69 w/o CC

See **DRG 096.**

DRG 098

MDC 04	RW$ 0.4275	Medical	Outlier Cutoff 11	Mean LOS 3.7

Bronchitis and Asthma – Age 0–17

PRINCIPAL DIAGNOSES WITH POTENTIAL HOME CARE NEEDS

Asthma
Bronchitis

DETAILS TO CONSIDER

Patient is under 18. Education of patient/caregiver is important to ensure compliance with health care regimen. The reader is referred to pediatric texts for additional information.

DRG 099

MDC 04	RW$ 0.8035	Medical	Outlier Cutoff 26	Mean LOS 5.5

Respiratory Signs and Symptoms – Age > = 70 and/or CC

PRINCIPAL DIAGNOSES WITH POTENTIAL HOME CARE NEEDS

Hiccough
Hemoptysis
Hyperventilation
Orthopnea

DETAILS TO CONSIDER

Patient is 70 or older with comorbidity and/or complications. Hyperventilation, orthopnea, hemoptysis, hiccough are manifestations of other health problems. Long-term follow-up is aimed at correcting causative factors (see appropriate DRG).

POTENTIAL HOME CARE PROBLEM

1. Knowledge deficit related to need for follow-up health care regimen.

PLAN

Instruct patient to notify physician regarding change in symptoms that may indicate other health problems.

DRG 100

MDC 04	RW$ 0.7730	Medical	Outlier Cutoff 24	Mean LOS 5.1

Respiratory Signs and Symptoms – Age < 70 w/o CC

See DRG 099.

MDC 04	RW$ 0.9035	Medical	Outlier Cutoff 27	Mean LOS 6.8

Other Respiratory Diagnoses – Age >= 70 and/or CC

PRINCIPAL DIAGNOSES WITH POTENTIAL HOME CARE NEEDS

Asphyxia
Foreign body in trachea, bronchus, lung
Pectus excavatum

DETAILS TO CONSIDER

Patient is 70 or older with comorbidity and/or complications.

POTENTIAL HOME CARE PROBLEMS	PLAN
1. Health management deficit secondary to patient's age and other illness.	Assess patient's ability to comply with health regime for other illness and follow-up care for present hospitalization. Assess impact of illness on ability to care for self.
2. Potential fluid volume deficit/overload secondary to cardiac complications if present.	Assess patient's fluid balance. Instruct in fluid restriction if indicated; daily weigh-in.
3. Potential alteration in nutrition.	Instruct in specified diet order.
4. Potential for ineffective breathing pattern.	Instruct patient in importance of cough and deep-breathing exercises. Encourage change in position and increased activity to promote maximum lung expansion. (Patient may tend to inhibit chest movement and use shallow breathing to avoid discomfort.)
5. Pain management.	Instruct in proper usage of analgesics. Have patient splint chest while coughing.
6. Knowledge deficit related to health care plan.	Instruct in correct usage of medications if ordered. Instruct patient to report unusual symptoms to physician (i.e. fever, increased sputum production, dyspnea).

MDC 04	RW$ 0.9024	Medical	Outlier Cutoff 26	Mean LOS 6.1

Other Respiratory Diagnoses – Age < 70

See **DRG 101**.

5 MDC 05
DISEASES AND DISORDERS OF THE CIRCULATORY SYSTEM

SURGICAL GROUPINGS (18 DRGs)

Heart Transplant

Cardiac Valve Procedure with Pump

Coronary Bypass

Cardiothoracic Procedures

Major Reconstructive Vascular Procedures

Vascular Procedures

Amputation for Circulatory System Disorders

Permanent Cardiac Pacemaker Implant

Cardiac Pacemaker Replacements and Revisions

Vein Ligation and Stripping

MEDICAL GROUPINGS (25 DRGs)

Circulatory Disorders

Acute and Subacute Endocarditis

Deep Vein Thrombosis

Heart Failure and Shock

Cardiac Arrest

Peripheral Vascular Disorders

Atherosclerosis

Hypertension

Cardiac Congenital and Valvular Disorders

Cardiac Arrhythmia and Conduction Disorders

Angina Pectoris

Syncope and Collapse

Chest Pain

Other Circulatory Diagnoses

MASTER HOME CARE PLANNING GUIDE
FOR CONDITIONS OF THE CIRCULATORY SYSTEM

Pattern	Assessment Factors	Plan
1. Health management deficit	Determine length of acute/chronic illness. Has patient become weak and unable to care for self/others? Has patient's employment been affected? Does patient require the intervention of mechanical support systems to maintain health status? Will the patient require long-term drug therapy, nutritional and activity alternatives in order to maintain health? What is the patient's/family's understanding of diagnosis/prognosis and what are their initial plans for adjustment based on diagnosis/prognosis?	Review previous diagnosis through conversations with health care team, patient and family. Early involvement with appropriate resources, i.e. social services, discharge planning, physical therapy, dietary, psychiatry, oncology, pharmacology and all other members of the health care team (doctors and nurses) for a multidisciplinary approach. Assessment of patient's ability to comply with medical follow-up based on potential need for medical therapy secondary to chronic disease process. Determine health care teaching needs appropriate to specific DRG.
1a. Potential for infection	Determine potential based on diagnosis and trends in prognosis. Will the patient require long-term immunosuppression due to implantation of artificial devices and/or foreign tissues? Will the patient require chronic long-term medical intervention due to potential complications which occur with diagnosis?	Assess patient/family need for teaching based on diagnosis/prognosis. Review of signs/symptoms of infection/rejection based on implantation and/or immunosuppression needs. Discuss precautions and changes significant to threat in health care maintenance.
2. Alteration in nutrition	Determine current nutritional status based on length of acute/chronic illness. Determine potential nutritional needs essential to promoting wound healing, general strengthening and maintenance of optimal activity levels. Investigate required dietary restrictions necessary to support alteration or arresting of disease process, lifestyle changes, and medication therapy.	Seek early dietary involvement to establish baseline nutritional statistics as well as progressive nutritional support. Determine paitent's ability to comply with potential nutritional restrictions. Determine dietary restrictions needed to support current and future health statistics to include precautions due to drug therapies, alteration in activity levels, and progressive disease processes.
2a. Potential impairment of skin integrity	Compromised cardiac and circulatory status directly affects perfusion to all body parts. Decreased circulation to organs and surface tissues can lead to long-term chronic problems which can include functional organ changes and dehydration, ulceration and necrosis to surface tissues.	Evaluate current organ function and surface tissue integrity. Identify current level of changes to include: alteration in sensation, temperature, capillary filling, pulses and discoloration or ulceration to surface tissues and peripheral limbs and digits. Determine level of wound healing.

3. Alteration in elimination

Alteration in circulation can lead to gastrointestinal and urological system changes. Long-term chronic changes can cause reduced function to bowel and kidney/bladder function. Long-term medication therapy (i.e. immunosuppression, anticoagulation therapy, etc.) can result in increased gastric acidity, gastrointestinal bleeding, alteration in glucose level control, renal function and urinary tract bleeding.

Establish baseline function of gastrointestinal and urological tract and current elimination patterns. Instruct patient in potential for alterations in gastrointestinal and urological tract based on current disease process. Instruct patient in assessment of future GI/GU tract function to include: signs/symptoms of impaired function, potential changes due to specific medication therapy and potential need to monitor for occult blood in stools, urine, sugar and acetones in urine, intake and output as determined by long-term therapy. Determine patient's level of ability to report all untoward changes.

4. Activity and exercise: potential for required change based on altered circulatory status

Assess level of home management deficit based on diagnosis as mild/moderate/severe or chronic. Assess need for use of adaptive equipment. Identify need for use of antiembolism garments. Assess need for alterations in activity patterns based on diagnosis/treatment prognosis.

Determine current level of functioning based on diagnosis. Determine potential for increased or decreased activity levels based on prognosis (early intervention by physical therapy). Instruct patient on projected activity, exercise program and limits based on diagnosis/prognosis. Instruct in use and care of required equipment. Discuss patient's alternatives in lifestyle changes.

4a. Home maintenance management deficit

Assess level of home management deficit based on prognosis and/or disease process.

Interview patient/family to determine living arrangements, support groups, bathroom facilities, structural layout concerns, equipment needs, grocery supplies, transportation for follow-up, homemaker needs and financial concerns. Early intervention is essential. Determine potential home management deficit considering: diagnosis/ prognosis, equipment needs, level of care needed, ability and availability of caregiver, and willingness of family members/friends to assist with home care maintenance.

5. Cognitive perceptual deficit — lack of knowledge related to self-care.	Assess patient's ability to understand diagnosis/prognosis. Assess patient's understanding of alterations in practices required to maintain current health status or alter future health changes. Determine teaching needs.	Determine what changes in lifestyle are required to support a healthful state. Instruct patient in all changes required to include: dietary activity, medical therapy, equipment use, job changes as indicated by diagnosis/prognosis. Assess patient's ability to comply with changes. Determine patient's willingness to follow future medical follow-up. Assess need for follow-up of home health care team to provide ongoing assessment of health care maintenance program.
5a. Pain management	Long-term circulatory impairment can lead to chronic exacerbations of pain due to neurological/vascular changes. Assess patient's pain threshold and plan for pain control through pain medication, comfort measures and diversional activities.	Discuss pain management with patient/family to include — use of medication therapy and potential problems with long-term narcotic use, techniques for comfort measures and plans for use of diversional activities and support groups.
6. Alteration in self-perception and increased anxiety	Diseases of the circulatory system can often lead to long-term hospitalization and/or recurrent admissions as well as chronic health care problems. Changes in employment status may occur. Long-term drug therapy can cause personality changes and emotional depression.	Investigate past patterns of self-perception and ability to deal with stress/anxiety. Encourage patient/family to verbalize concerns and fears. Seek appropriate counseling based on identified needs (early involvement of social services needed in cases of financial concerns).
6a. Body image disturbances	Alterations in self-perception can occur due to patient's psychological reaction to the need for implantation of foreign tissues/mechanical parts and/or loss of body parts.	Assess patient's/family's reaction to altered physical status and allow verbalization of fears/thoughts (seek appropriate counseling as indicated). Provide accurate information about the purpose/function of indwelling mechanical or tissue parts (see specific DRGs).

7.	Role relationship: dependent/independent status — potential for conflict	The disabling effects of heart disease often lead to alterations in self-care management, employment ability, and dependent/independent roles. Prognosis of future chronic problems compound potential conflicts in role changes.	Determine current level of function and future potential changes. Discuss potential for future changes and determine their plans for coping with role changes. Seek appropriate counseling as indicated.
8.	Sexuality — sexual dysfunction	Alteration in physical tolerance to sexual activity can occur in progressive circulatory diseases. Subsequent changes can cause stress to marital relationships.	Discuss potential need for alteration in sexual activity based on disease process — seek appropriate counseling when indicated. Evaluate patient's/family's ability to cope with discussion and instruction on required changes and encourage patient/family to verbalize their anxiety/concerns and questions.
9.	Coping tolerance	Long-term prognosis, length of hospitalization and patient's ability to deal with responsibility will affect patient's ability to cope with disease process.	Communicate known factors about recuperative phase and/or long-term effects of disease process/prognosis. Seek appropriate counseling where indicated (specific to age group concerns).

DRG 103

Heart Transplant

*No values have been established for this DRG.

OPERATIVE PROCEDURE WITH POTENTIAL HOME CARE NEEDS

Heart transplant

DETAILS TO CONSIDER

Patients undergoing heart transplantation have had end-stage cardiac disease with poor prognosis for survival prior to transplantation. Criteria for transplant include healthy general status other than end-stage cardiac disease.

POTENTIAL HOME CARE PROBLEMS	PLAN
1. Health management deficit — related to need for long-term medical treatment.	Assess patient's understanding of need for follow-up medical treatment to include: routine EKG, chest x-ray, lab work and endomyocardial biopsies. Assess patient's understanding of lifelong medication therapy to include: dosage, action, expected effects, side effects. Assess patient's understanding of need for strict monitoring for signs of rejection to include: weight gain, peripheral edema, increased jugular pulsation, malaise, fever and sensory changes as well as imbalance in intake and output.
1a. Potential for infection secondary to immunosuppression therapy.	Instruct patient in signs of infection to include: fever, malaise, upper respiratory infection, urinary tract infection, fungal infections and increased sensitivity to mucous membranes. Establish record for monitoring temperature changes.
2. Alteration in nutrition secondary to atherosclerotic risk factor and drug-induced glucose level changes.	Determine dietary requirements/restrictions (early dietary assessment essential). Instruct patient in dietary restrictions to include: weight control, sodium restrictions, modified fat and sugar content and potential fluid restrictions.
3. Elimination problems secondary to altered diet, change in activity levels, and medication side effects.	Instruct patient in regime for monitoring changes in GI function, increased gastric acidity, occult stool, sugar and acetone, weigh daily, check to monitor fluid retention, increase in peripheral edema and imbalances in intake and output.
4. Potential need for activity program secondary to muscle wasting and immunosuppression therapy.	See **Master Care Plan.** Instruct patient in progressive activity program to prevent muscle wasting and bone/joint involvement secondary to long-term immunosuppression therapy.

5. Cognitive/perceptual deficit — knowledge deficit related to self-care.

Instruct patient in need for independent management of medication schedules, dietary restrictions, activity program, monitoring for potential infections and signs of rejection to include: weight gain, peripheral edema, increase in jugular vein pulsation, malaise, fever and sensorium changes.

6. Self-perception — potential for depression/personality changes secondary to drug therapy and altered lifestyle.

Instruct patient/family in medication side effects which may include emotional depression, personality changes. Encourage verbalization about reactions to adherence to specific lifestyle changes.

REFERRAL INFORMATION

Dependent upon individual needs. Most patients are followed by a transplant team.

DRG 104

| MDC 05 | RW$ 6.8527 | Surgical | Outlier Cutoff 41 | Mean LOS 20.9 |

Cardiac Valve Procedure with Pump and Cardiac Catheter

OPERATIVE PROCEDURES WITH POTENTIAL HOME CARE NEEDS

Mitral valve replacement
Atrial valve replacement
Valve replacement with cardiac catheter done on same admission

DETAILS TO CONSIDER

Rheumatic fever is one of the leading causes of valvular disease. The patient with valvular disease may have had long-term problems with pulmonary edema, pulmonary hypertension, congestive heart failure, cardiac arrhythmias (atrial fibrillation and atrial flutter), peripheral edema and compromised renal function.

POTENTIAL HOME CARE PROBLEMS

PLAN

1. Health management deficit related to need for long-term medical therapy.

Assess patient's understanding of long-term therapy to include medication and continued treatment for presurgical conditions. Determine patient's need for anticoagulation therapy and instruct patient on dosage, potential need for frequent adjustment of medication based on lab work and potential complications from anticoagulant therapy to include signs/symptoms of "over" anticoagulation states and precautions to be used while on anticoagulants.

1a. Potential for infection.

Assess wound healing. Instruct patient in signs/symptoms of infection at incision and catheterization sites.

2.	Alteration in nutrition secondary to drug therapies and/or cardiac disease status.	Determine dietary restrictions required and instruct patient (often include sodium, cholesterol restrictions). Instruct in restrictions on vitamin K foods in cases of anticoagulation therapy (instruct in fluid restrictions as indicated).
3.	Elimination problems secondary to dietary restrictions, altered activity levels and/or medication side effects.	Instruct patient in monitoring for adequate elimination function, signs/symptoms of fluid retention and internal bleeding due to anticoagulation therapy.
4.	Alteration in activity based on cardiac status.	See **Master Care Plan** (review activity percautions if anticoagulation therapy is indicated). Teach assessment of limb involved in cardiac catheterization to include: color, temperature, sensation, pulses, and wound healing.
5.	Cognitive deficit potential for memory defect secondary to cerebral hypoxia and/or pain medication effect.	Evaluate neuro status. Explain potential for short-term memory loss (medication-affected) and precautions to use in providing a safe environment in cases of depressed nervous status. Review measures for pain relief to reduce narcotic use.
6.	Self-perception, potential for body image disturbances secondary to patient's reaction to implantation of mechanical or porcine valve.	See **Master Care Plan** (instruct patient/family on potential for hearing "click" when mechanical valve used).

REFERRAL INFORMATION

Referral to home care nurse will depend on patient's ability to carry out activities of daily living. Patient may participate in cardiac rehabilitation program after discharge.

DRG 105

MDC 05	RW$ 5.2308	Surgical	Outlier Cutoff 36	Mean LOS 16.2

Cardiac Valve Procedure with Pump and w/o Cardiac Catheter

OPERATIVE PROCEDURES WITH POTENTIAL HOME CARE NEEDS

Same as **DRG 104** but without cardiac catheter on same admission.

MDC 05   **RW$ 5.2624**   **Surgical**   **Outlier Cutoff 40**   **Mean LOS 20.4**

Coronary Bypass with Cardiac Catheter

OPERATIVE PROCEDURES WITH POTENTIAL HOME CARE NEEDS

Aortocoronary bypass
Internal mammary artery bypass with cardiac catheter done on same admission

DETAILS TO CONSIDER

Coronary artery disease develops due to obstructed atherosclerotic changes in the branches of the coronary arteries. Patients requiring coronary artery bypass may have underlying disease states which range from chronic disabling angina pectoris to acute myocardial infarction with extension and anginal pain that is nonresponsive to medication. Peripheral vascular disease, cardiac arrhythmias, increased blood pressure, and decreased renal function may also be indicated from previous diagnoses.

POTENTIAL HOME CARE PROBLEMS	PLAN
1. Health management deficit related to long-term medical diagnosis.	Assess patient's understanding of medical diagnosis and possible long-term medication therapy secondary to prebypass history.
1a. Potential for wound infection.	See **DRG 104** (section on wound infection).
2. Alteration in nutrition intake secondary to atherosclerotic changes.	See **Master Care Plan** (nutrition section).
2a. Skin integrity — potential impairment due to decreased blood supply secondary to removal of saphenous or cephalic veins.	See **Master Care Plan.** Instruct patient in use of nonrestrictive clothing on limb involved. Instruct patient in avoidance of position that could hinder blood flow to limb involved (crossing legs, sitting for long periods).

REFERRAL INFORMATION

Same as **DRG 104.**

MDC 05   **RW$ 3.9891**   **Surgical**   **Outlier Cutoff 34**   **Mean LOS 13.5**

Coronary Bypass w/o Cardiac Catheter

OPERATIVE PROCEDURES WITH POTENTIAL HOME CARE NEEDS

Aortocoronary bypass
Internal mammary coronary bypass without cardiac catheter on same admission.

See **DRG 106** and delete any discussion related to cardiac catheterization follow-up.

DRG 108

MDC 05	RW$ 4.3756	Surgical	Outlier Cutoff 33	Mean LOS 13.3

Cardiothoracic Procedure, Except Valve and Coronary Bypass, with Pump

OPERATIVE PROCEDURES WITH POTENTIAL HOME CARE NEEDS

Heart septa repair
Heart aneurysm excision
Total repair, tetralogy of Fallot
Total repair, truncus arteriosus

DETAILS TO CONSIDER

Congenital anomalies present in three major hemodynamic pattern changes: volume overload, pressure overload and devastation of circulating arterial blood. Surgical repairs are based on the specific correction of the defect(s) causing the hemodynamic change(s). Medical management also is prescribed based on the signs/symptoms of the defect(s). Potential home care problems are based not only on the patient but also on the family members who must care for the child or young adult with the effects of these defects.

REFERRAL INFORMATION

Background information — communicate health status and pertinent patient/parent/family situations and living situations. Current hospitalization/complications — course of illness, current status, complications, parental reaction to defects and identified ability to cope with health care management of child/young adult with anomalies.

DRG 109

MDC 05	RW$ 3.6963	Surgical	Outlier Cutoff 32	Mean LOS 12.1

Cardiothoracic Procedures w/o Pump

OPERATIVE PROCEDURES WITH POTENTIAL HOME CARE NEEDS

Closed valvotomy
Pericardiectomy

DETAILS TO CONSIDER

Patients requiring valvotomy or pericardiectomy have long-standing history of cardiac disease in process. Long-term needs are dependent on the individual's cardiac history, chronic disease state and long-term prognosis.

See **DRGs 104** and **106.**

MDC 05   **RW$ 2.9328**   **Surgical**   **Outlier Cutoff 34**   **Mean LOS 14.3**

Major Reconstructive Vascular Procedures – Age > = 70 and/or CC

OPERATIVE PROCEDURES WITH POTENTIAL HOME CARE NEEDS

Aorta resection with replacement
Aorta aneurysm repair
Leg artery resection with anastomosis

DETAILS TO CONSIDER

Long-term need dependent on patient's previous diagnosis and chronic disease status caused by complications. All reconstructive vascular procedures have potential to cause chronic circulatory compromise.

POTENTIAL HOME CARE PROBLEM

Tissue perfusion — potential for compromised circulatory function.

PLAN

Assess tissue perfusion distal to area of resection (to include superficial tissue as well as organ perfusion). Instruct patient in assessment of perfusion to include changes in color, temperature, capillary fill, pulses, sensation and ulcerations. Instruct in GI/GU function and potential changes due to complications resulting from circulatory compromise. Determine need for evaluation of mental acuity. Determine need for anti-coagulation therapy. Give instruction as indicated.

DRG 111

MDC 05   **RW$ 2.5851**   **Surgical**   **Outlier Cutoff 33**   **Mean LOS 13.2**

Major Reconstructive Vascular Procedures – Age < 70 w/o CC

See **DRG 110.**

DRG 112

Vascular Procedures Except Major Reconstruction

OPERATIVE PROCEDURES WITH POTENTIAL HOME CARE NEEDS

Endarterectomy
Plication of vena cava
Clipping of aneurysm

DETAILS TO CONSIDER

There is potential for dislodgment of plaque(s) or thrombus, which can result in an embolic effect.

POTENTIAL HOME CARE NEEDS	PLAN
1. Health management deficit related to need for long-term medical follow-up.	Review need for blood pressure control with drug usage and/or dietary restrictions.
2. Alteration in nutrition.	Determine dietary restrictions and changes based on medical history and recommendations of physician. Instruct patient/family in dietary changes. If anticoagulation therapy is indicated instruct in dietary restrictions concerning foods high in vitamin K.
3. Activity/exercise pattern — potential for alteration in tissue perfusion secondary to surgical procedure and/or postoperative complications of emboli.	Review activity restrictions if indicated. Instruct patient/family in signs and symptoms of neurological dysfunction secondary to cerebral ischemia or emboli as well as potential respiratory complications secondary to emboli formation.
4. Cognitive/perceptive knowledge deficit.	Review potential for recurrent cardiovascular and cerebrovascular disease based on progressive atherosclerotic changes.

REFERRAL INFORMATION

See **DRG 106.**

Amputation for Circulatory System Disorders Except Upper Limb and Toe

OPERATIVE PROCEDURES WITH POTENTIAL HOME CARE NEEDS

Lower limb amputation
Below-knee amputation
Above-knee amputation
Disarticulation of hip
Hind-quarter disarticulation

DETAILS TO CONSIDER

Patient undergoing amputation of limb due to circulatory compromise will have underlying chronic disease states. Comorbidity diagnoses may increase long-term needs. Diabetes (**DRGs 294** and **295**), Peripheral Vascular Disorders (**DRGs 130** and **131**), and Deep Vein Thrombosis (**DRG 128**).

POTENTIAL HOME CARE PROBLEMS

PLAN

1. Health management deficit — potential related to long-term medical therapy.

Assess patient's understanding and potential for compliance with follow-up treatment. Assess patient's understanding of disease process and long-term prognosis. Involve patient/family early in discussion of postoperative course and plans for rehabilitation.

2. Alteration in nutritional pattern to promote stump healing while maintaining optimum weight.

Instruct patient in nutritional requirements needed to promote wound healing while maintaining optimum weight.

3. Activity/exercise program secondary to loss of limb and potential for contractures, difficulty with ambulation and potential prosthetic use.

(Early physical therapy involvement). Refer to physical therapy program to prevent contractures and to strengthen other body parts essential in maintaining optimum mobility and preparation for prosthesis.

4. Self-perception — body image disturbance.

Foster environment conducive to patient's discussion about reaction/feelings toward loss of body part. Evaluate patient's ability to comply with rigorous therapy program.

REFERRAL INFORMATION

Background information — pertinent health history and prognosis, pertinent family situation and living arrangements, potential for prosthetic replacement. Current hospital history — including complications. Course of illness, patient progress in active physical therapy program and ability to do activities of daily living, physiological reaction to loss of body part. Durable medical equipment — depending upon living facilities, investigate for temporary need of wheelchair, commode, hospital bed, trapeze, crutches, walker, sliding board and eventual fitting of prosthesis. Will need community contacts that can assist in alterations in transportation vehicles to facilitate driving with lower limb handicap.

DRG 114

MDC 05	RW$ 2.1067	Surgical	Outlier Cutoff 37	Mean LOS 16.6

Upper Limb and Toe Amputation for Circulatory System Disorders

OPERATIVE PROCEDURES WITH POTENTIAL HOME CARE NEEDS

Amputation of finger, hand, forearm
Shoulder disarticulation
Toe amputation
Amputation stump revision

DETAILS TO CONSIDER

See **DRG 113.**

Also include potential need for equipment to assist in activities of daily living as well as alteration in transportation vehicles to facilitate driving with upper limb handicap.

DRG 115

MDC 05	RW$ 3.9150	Surgical	Outlier Cutoff 36	Mean LOS 15.8

Permanent Cardiac Pacemaker Implant with AMI or CHF

OPERATIVE PROCEDURES WITH POTENTIAL HOME CARE NEEDS

Permanent cardiac pacemaker implant with AMI or CHF.

DETAILS TO CONSIDER

Comorbidity diagnoses which may increase long-term needs are:
   AMI — acute myocardial infarction (**DRG 121 and 122**)
   CHF — congestive heart failure (**DRG 127**)

POTENTIAL HOME CARE PROBLEMS	PLAN
1. Health management deficit secondary to need for long-term medical follow-up.	Assess patient's/family's ability to comply with medical follow-up based on long-term needs resulting from AMI, CHF and need for permanent pacer.
1a. Potential for infection at pacer insertion site.	Instruct patient/family in signs and symptoms of wound healing infections and allergy to foreign material. Monitor wound healing.
2. Potential alteration in nutritional pattern.	Determine dietary restrictions with physician based on medical history. Instruct patient and family in restrictions.
3. Alteration in activity and exercise pattern.	Determine activity/exercise program pertinent to individual patient. Instruct patient/family in need for a progressive activity program.

4. Cognitive/perceptual deficit — lack of knowledge about function of permanent pacemaker.

Instruct patient/family in purpose and function or malfunction of pacemaker to include monitoring of own pulse and maintaining a written record, knowledge of acceptable variations for own pacemaker as well as need to report episodes of chest pain, blackouts, syncope. Explain need for periodic pacemaker checks on function of pacer and potential need for battery charges at 1–3 year intervals depending on the model of pacemaker. Instruct patient in precautions against close proximity to high-frequency electronic equipment such as microwave ovens, engines, mowers, and snowmobiles. Instruct in need for reporting to all health professionals the presence of an implanted pacemaker prior to receiving any medical attention. Patient should carry ID card about pacemaker and/or use a medical alert bracelet and maintain a permanent record of make, model and serial number of the pacemaker and the frequency of replacement needs. A booklet is usually provided to the patient at the time of implantation with this information.

DRG 116

MDC 05	RW$ 2.8665	Surgical	Outlier Cutoff 29	Mean LOS 9.3

Permanent Cardiac Pacemaker Implant w/o AMI or CHF

OPERATIVE PROCEDURE WITH POTENTIAL HOME CARE NEEDS

Permanent cardiac pacemaker implant w/o AMI or CHF

See **DRG 115** but exclude information about AMI or CHF.

DRG 117

MDC 05	RW$ 1.8210	Surgical	Outlier Cutoff 26	Mean LOS 6.4

Cardiac Pacemaker Replacement and Revision Excluding Pulse Generation Replacement Only

OPERATIVE PROCEDURES WITH POTENTIAL HOME CARE NEEDS

Replacement of pacemaker electrodes
Remove pacemaker system

See **DRG 115.**

DRG 118

MDC 05	RW$ 1.7809	Surgical	Outlier Cutoff 18	Mean LOS 4.2

Cardiac Pacemaker Pulse Generator Replacement Only

OPERATIVE PROCEDURE WITH POTENTIAL HOME CARE NEEDS

Cardiac pacemaker pulse generator replacement only

See **DRGs 115** and **116.**

DRG 119

MDC 05	RW$ 1.0610	Surgical	Outlier Cutoff 27	Mean LOS 7.2

Vein Ligation and Stripping

OPERATIVE PROCEDURE WITH POTENTIAL HOME CARE NEEDS

Vein ligation and stripping of leg or arm

DETAILS TO CONSIDER

Comorbidity diagnoses which may increase long-term needs include:
    Diabetes (**DRG 294** and **295**).
    Circulatory System (**DRG 128, 130** and **131**).

POTENTIAL HOME CARE PROBLEMS

1. Health perception deficit — lack of knowledge about need for routine medical follow-up.

2. Cognitive/perceptual pattern — lacks knowledge about discharge regime to be followed.

PLAN

Assess patient's understanding of and compliance with routine medical follow-up.

Teach patient/family about need to follow regime that promotes venous return and prevents venous stress to include: avoidance of restrictive clothing (i.e. girdles, garters, tight elastic sleeves) leg crossing or standing for long periods or prolonged flexion of arm, use of support stockings or panty hose or support sleeves as prescribed by physician and routine elevation of affected limbs to promote venous return. Also instruct patient in need for ambulation for 5 minutes each hour during periods of prolonged sitting and need for progressive ambulation up to 40 minutes daily. Instruct patient in signs/symptoms of phlebitis and changes in loss of skin on affected limbs and need for reporting changes quickly.

Other Operating Room Procedures of the Circulatory System

OPERATIVE PROCEDURES WITH POTENTIAL HOME CARE NEEDS

Dialysis arteriovenostomy
Revision of shunt

DETAILS TO CONSIDER

Comorbidity diagnoses which may increase long-term needs include:
Circulatory (DRGs 127, 128, 130 and 132).
Renal failure (DRGs 316 and 317).

POTENTIAL HOME CARE PROBLEMS

1. Health perception management deficit — lack of knowledge about long-term medical needs.

1a. Cognitive/perceptual pattern — lack of knowledge about care and precautions of shunt/fistula to ensure patency.

2. Self-perception — body image disturbance.

PLAN

Determine patient's understanding of diagnosis/prognosis and long-term need for hemodialysis. Determine patient's compliance potential toward long-term medical treatment and alterations in lifestyle due to chronic hemodialysis. Instruct patient in potential need for frequent shunt/fistula revisions.

Instruct patient in precautions and care of fistula/shunt to include:

- length of time needed for AV fistula maturation.
- use of enteral shunt in interim.
- potential for aneurysm formation signs and symptoms.
- care of shunt or fistula site.
- limitations on length of use of a shunt.
- dislodgment or hemorrhage potential — instruct in proper application of clips in cases of shunt separation.
- precautions regarding affected limbs such as avoidance of restrictive clothing.
- how to assess for fistula/shunt patency such as pulse-taking and checking for decreased circulation to involved limb.
- patient should be instructed to obtain a medical alert bracelet.

Encourage open discussion about patient's concerns and feelings regarding chronic dialysis and presence of a visible reminder of his/her disease and chronic dependence on a machine.

DRG 121

MDC 05	RW$ 1.8648	Medical	Outlier Cutoff 32	Mean LOS 11.9

Circulatory Disorders with AMI and Cardiovascular Complications — Discharged Alive

PRINCIPAL DIAGNOSES WITH POTENTIAL HOME CARE NEEDS

Acute myocardial infarction and cardiovascular complications
Malignant hypertension, heart disease with congestive heart failure
Heart block
Heart failure
Dissecting aneurysm

DETAILS TO CONSIDER

See Circulatory DRGs 132–134.

POTENTIAL HOME CARE PROBLEMS

PLAN

1. Health perception management — knowledge deficit related to disease process/prognosis.

Assess patient's/family's understanding of and compliance with long-term chronic disease process and need for routine medical treatment.

2. Potential for cognitive improvement — lack of knowledge about routines, lifestyle changes needed.

Instruct patient in disease process and prognosis — potential for cardiac healing process post-MI and/or extension of disease, medication, diet, activity requirements. Evaluate adaptability compliance to lifestyle changes and coping techniques for dealing with stress. Instruct in signs and symptoms of disease progression and need to report changes quickly. Instruct patient in use of blood pressure equipment to facilitate frequent monitoring of blood pressure.

3. Self-perception — body image disturbances.

Assess patient's/family's ability to express their concerns and feelings about loss of previous body functioning, job capability and usual role in the family. Help patient and family to make tentative plan for modifying lifestyle to adjust to current disease status.

DRG 122

MDC 05	RW$ 1.3651	Medical	Outlier Cutoff 30	Mean LOS 9.8

Circulatory Disorders with AMI w/o Cardiovascular Complications — Discharged Alive

PRINCIPAL DIAGNOSIS WITH POTENTIAL HOME CARE NEEDS

Acute myocardial infarction with any other diagnosis of circulatory disorder.

See DRG 121.

MDC 05   **RW$ 1.1360**   **Medical**   **Outlier Cutoff 23**   **Mean LOS 3.1**

Circulatory Disorders with AMI — Expired

No home care needs for patient. Follow-up care for family should be arranged through social services, clergy or family physician.

MDC 05   **RW$ 2.2200**   **Medical**   **Outlier Cutoff 28**   **Mean LOS 8.4**

Circulatory Disorders Except AMI with Cardiac Catheter and Complex Diagnosis

PRINCIPAL DIAGNOSES WITH POTENTIAL HOME CARE NEEDS

Myocarditis
Endocarditis
Cardiomyopathy

All with cardiac catheter on same admission.

DETAILS TO CONSIDER

Cardiomyopathy represents a primary disease that affects the ventricular muscle rather than a secondary disease resulting from other cardiac abnormalities. Home care planning needs are based on the individual complications presented in each case which can include congestive heart failure, arrhythmias and systemic or pulmonic thromboembolic states.

POTENTIAL HOME CARE PROBLEMS

1. Health perception and management deficits secondary to knowledge deficit about potential chronic progressive disease state.

2. Cognitive and perceptual deficit secondary to lack of knowledge re: medication, activity, nutritional routines to be followed.

PLAN

Assess patient/family understanding of disease process and need for strict medical follow-up on routine basis.

Assess patient/family ability to comply with specific medication routine. Instruct patient in usage of medication, dose frequency, expected effect and side effects. Condition is frequently treated with diuretics, antiarrhythmia drugs, potassium supplements and long-term anticoagulation medicines. Discuss need for routine medical follow-up to include:
- EKG
- chest x-ray and lab work.

Instruct in dietary restrictions and any concerns pertinent to individual case. Review activity levels and lifestyle changes as disease process dictates.

DRG 125

Circulatory Disorders Except AMI
with Cardiac Catheter w/o Complex Diagnosis

PRINCIPAL DIAGNOSES WITH POTENTIAL HOME CARE NEEDS

Cardiac catheterization
Angiocardiogram
Arteriogram

DETAILS TO CONSIDER

The patient requiring cardiac catheterization has already experienced health changes that have indicated cardiac disease. Home care planning should focus on wound healing at catheter insertion site and assisting patient/family to cope with outcome and recommended course of action.

POTENTIAL HOME CARE PROBLEMS

1. Health perception and management — potential for infection at catheter site.

2. Cognitive/perceptual pattern — knowledge deficit of disease process.

PLAN

Instruct patient and family in routine process for wound healing to include:
- signs and symptoms of infection or phlebitis.
- potential for development of aneurysm at insertion site.
- inspection for changes in circulation to affected limb.

Confirm follow-up medical care for removal of sutures and inspection of wound. Have patient demonstrate proper technique for care of wound and inspection for adequate circulation.

Assess patient's understanding and acceptance of diagnostic outcome and knowledge of course of action.

MDC 05   **RW$ 2.6645**   **Medical**   **Outlier Cutoff 38**   **Mean LOS 18.4**

Acute and Subacute Endocarditis

PRINCIPAL DIAGNOSES WITH POTENTIAL HOME CARE NEEDS

Acute endocarditis
Subacute endocarditis

DETAILS TO CONSIDER

Home care planning for endocarditis is dependent on complications resulting from the inflammatory process. Most common complications are congenital heart failure and valvular insufficiency.

See DRGs related to potential circulatory complications (**104, 105, 124, 127**).

MDC 05   **RW$ 1.0408**   **Medical**   **Outlier Cutoff 28**   **Mean LOS 7.8**

Heart Failure and Shock

PRINCIPAL DIAGNOSES WITH POTENTIAL HOME CARE NEEDS

Rheumatic heart failure
Congestive heart failure (CHF)

DETAILS TO CONSIDER

The focus for home care planning in heart failure is to ensure patient understanding of measures needed to restore adequate cardiac output through increased efficiency of myocardial contractions. Adherence to such measures is essential to avoid secondary problems from inadequate organ perfusion to such areas as renal, pulmonary or cerebral systems.

POTENTIAL HOME CARE PROBLEMS

1. Health perception/management — knowledge deficit regarding disease process and potential complications.

2. Cognitive and perceptual pattern — knowledge deficit.

PLAN

Assess patient's understanding of disease process and treatment plans to reduce work load of heart. Instruction to include medication therapy along with rest, digitalization, diuretics and diet restrictions.

Instruct patient in basic facts of CHF to include signs and symptoms, treatment and preventive measures for recurrent attacks. Also include activity restrictions, diet changes, medication effects and side effects.

EQUIPMENT NEEDS

Dependent upon home situation. May require oxygen therapy in home.

DRG 128

MDC 05   **RW$ 0.8639**   **Medical**   **Outlier Cutoff 28**   **Mean LOS 9.6**

Deep Vein Thrombosis

DIAGNOSIS WITH POTENTIAL HOME CARE NEEDS

Deep vein thrombosis (DVT)

DETAILS TO CONSIDER

Postphlebitic syndrome with chronic stasis can occur as a residual effect of phlebitis. Specific detail to prevention measures is essential.

POTENTIAL HOME CARE PROBLEMS	PLAN
1. Health perception and management — knowledge deficit regarding cause and effects of deep vein thrombosis.	Review basic circulation function with patient. Explain alterations in circulation caused by DVT. Assess patient's understanding of medical treatment and review importance of adherence to medical regime in order to prevent recurrence and development of chronic venous stasis.
2. Nutritional/metabolic pattern — alteration in dietary pattern.	Review importance of adequate nutritional status and hydration. Review dietary restrictions for prevention of edema and maintenance of optimal body weight.
2a. Alteration in skin integrity.	Instruct patient in technique for inspection of skin to include evaluation of circulation, color, skin tone, edema, changes in sensation and identification of symptoms of recurrent phlebitis.
3. Elimination pattern — potential for GI/GU bleeding secondary to anticoagulation therapy.	Instruct patient in signs and symptoms of potential GI/GU bleeding due to over-coagulation therapy.
4. Activity restrictions secondary to compromise in circulation.	Instruct patient to elevate legs at least 5 inches above the level of heart by lying down 2–3 hours daily and at night to allow venous draining by gravity. Use of elastic stockings to prevent edema and instruct in the care of the garment. Avoid standing or sitting for prolonged periods. Avoid use of restrictive clothing and avoid activities that will increase chances of injury.
5. Cognitive/perceptual deficit — lack of knowledge about anticoagulation therapy.	Patient will demonstrate understanding of anticoagulation therapy to include drug dosage, expected effects, untoward effects and precautions for use, dietary and activity restrictions, frequency of blood tests, limits in use of other nonprescribed medications and use of medical alert bracelet. Instruct in signs/symptoms of recurrence of DVT and/or pulmonary embolus.
5a. Pain control — potential for chronic pain due to compromised circulation.	Instruct patient in use of narcotics for chronic pain control and in alternative measures for pain control.

| MDC 05 | RW$ 1.5506 | Medical | Outlier Cutoff 25 | Mean LOS 4.6 |

Cardiac Arrest

Instantaneous death.
Death within 24 hours of symptoms.

Follow-up support for family through clergy, social services and family physician.

| MDC 05 | RW$ 0.9645 | Medical | Outlier Cutoff 27 | Mean LOS 7.1 |

Peripheral Vascular Disorders – Age > = 70 and/or CC

PRINCIPAL DIAGNOSES WITH POTENTIAL HOME CARE NEEDS

Aneurysm
Arterial embolism
Superficial phlebitis
Leg varicosity with ulcer

DETAILS TO CONSIDER

See Circulatory **DRGs** (**128** plus **108**, **110** and **112**).

| MDC 05 | RW$ 0.9491 | Medical | Outlier Cutoff 26 | Mean LOS 6.4 |

Peripheral Vascular Disorders – Age < 70 w/o CC

See **DRGs 128** and **130**.

DRG 132

MDC 05   **RW$ 0.9182**   **Medical**   **Outlier Cutoff 27**   **Mean LOS 6.7**

Atherosclerosis – Age > = 70 and/or CC

PRINCIPAL DIAGNOSES WITH POTENTIAL HOME CARE NEEDS

Arteriosclerotic cardiovascular disease (ASCVD)
Cardiomegaly
Coronary atherosclerosis

DETAILS TO CONSIDER

Atherosclerosis is characterized by the accumulation of lipids and fibrous tissue in the wall of the artery causing subsequent obstructions. Such changes can lead to significant coronary disease and the complications that follow are numerous.

See Circulatory **DRGs (106, 107, 110, 112)**.

POTENTIAL HOME CARE PROBLEMS

1. Health perception/management deficit — related to risk factors.

2. Nutrition — alteration in current dietary habits in order to regain and maintain optimal weight and lower cholesterol and/or lipid level.

3. Activity/exercise — potential need for alteration in activity levels.

4. Cognitive/perceptual patterns — knowledge deficit regarding disease process.

PLAN

Assess patient's understanding of risk factors which contribute to the development and progression of atherosclerotic changes to include age, sex, family history, smoking, diet, hypertension, obesity, diabetes mellitus and personality type. Evaluate patient's willingness to comply with alternative in lifestyle based on individual's specific risk factors.

Obtain dietary consult early to begin diet development that will consider need for weight control, lipid level, cholesterol level and sugar/sweets restrictions.

Instruct in required alteration to support health status (may need to increase activity levels to prevent future complications or may need to decrease levels in patients who experience angina pectoris, peripheral vascular changes or edema).

Discuss potential for development of angina pectoris and/or myocardial infarction to include signs/symptoms of angina. Discuss potential need for coronary bypass dependent upon disease progression.

REFERRAL INFORMATION

Background information — significant health history and pertinent family/living situations. Current hospitalization/complications — course of illness, current status of complications and new restrictions to be maintained based on diagnosis/complications.

| MDC 05 | RW$ 0.8599 | Medical | Outlier Cutoff 25 | Mean LOS 5.2 |

Atherosclerosis – Age < 70 w/o CC

Same as **DRG 132.**

See Circulatory **DRGs (106, 107, 110, 112, 132).**

| MDC 05 | RW$ 0.7049 | Medical | Outlier Cutoff 26 | Mean LOS 6.1 |

Hypertension

PRINCIPAL DIAGNOSES WITH POTENTIAL HOME CARE NEEDS

Malignant hypertension with/without renal disease
Benign hypertension with/without renal disease

DETAILS TO CONSIDER

Treatment for hypertension varies depending on the diagnosis as primary (essential), secondary or accelerated (malignant).

POTENTIAL HOME CARE PROBLEMS

1. Nutrition — alteration in diet to support antihypertension therapy.

2. Activity/exercise — potential need for structured increased exercise program.

PLAN

Instruct patient in individualized diet routine to control weight, restrict fluid retention, reduce sodium consumption and reduce cholesterol and/or triglyceride levels.

Discuss when an increase in exercise is required. Review specifics to include gradual addition of exercises, duration and slow progressive increases in strenuousness of activity. Review signs/symptoms of sudden increase in blood pressure and/or angina pain.

3. Cognitive/perceptual deficit — lack of knowledge about disease process and prognosis.

Review known factors contributing to patient's hypertension (i.e. renal pathology, age, weight, race, smoking and dietary habits, activity levels, stress). Describe specific classifications of hypertension to patient with signs/symptoms to be expected and changes that can occur with compliant follow-through to medical regime. Review dietary activity and medication pattern to be used. Teach patient to monitor own blood pressure (sitting/standing) and maintain a record of findings — review signs and symptoms of sudden change in blood pressure (hypertension or hypotension) and when to report changes to physician.

REFERRAL INFORMATION

See **DRG 132.**

Monitor blood pressure of patient and instruct patient and family in independent monitoring of blood pressure. Equipment needs — blood pressure cuff, stethoscope and record book.

DRG 135

MDC 05	RW$ 0.9922	Medical	Outlier Cutoff 26	Mean LOS 6.1

Cardiac Congenital and Valvular Disorders – Age > = 70 and or CC

PRINCIPAL DIAGNOSIS WITH POTENTIAL HOME CARE NEEDS

Cardiac congenital and valvular disorders

DETAILS TO CONSIDER

See Circulatory **DRGs (104, 105, 108, 121,** and **127).**

DRG 136

MDC 05	RW$ 0.9674	Medical	Outlier Cutoff 25	Mean LOS 4.9

Cardiac Congenital and Valvular Disorders – Age 18–69 w/o CC

PRINCIPAL DIAGNOSIS WITH POTENTIAL HOME CARE NEEDS

Cardiac congenital and valvular disorders

DETAILS TO CONSIDER

See Circulatory **DRGs (104, 105, 108, 121,** and **127).**

MDC 05　　　**RW$ 0.6381**　　　**Medical**　　　**Outlier Cutoff 20**　　　**Mean LOS 3.3**

Cardiac Congenital and Valvular Disorders – Age 0–17

PRINCIPAL DIAGNOSIS WITH POTENTIAL HOME CARE NEEDS

Cardiac congenital and valvular disorders
Note *medical* admission vs admission for repair of anomaly.

DETAILS TO CONSIDER

See Circulatory **DRGs** (108, 127, 132, 134).

Children suffering from congenital anomalies may require frequent admissions for medical support for complications caused by the hemodynamic changes that occur with specific defects. Common complications include CHF, pulmonary infections and pulmonary edema. Medical care during these periods is aimed at the acute situation with frequent assessment toward potential complications.

POTENTIAL HOME CARE PROBLEMS	PLAN
1. Health perception/management deficit — related to prognosis.	Assess child's ability to understand simple explanations of current health status and future complications. Instructions or directions must be based on the age and maturity of the child. Parents must be instructed in current health status/complication management and estimations about future needs and potential prognosis.
2. Nutrition — alteration in dietary habits to support maintenance of optimal weight and nutritional balance.	Assess current dietary pattern in an effort to determine best feeding pattern for child (i.e. small frequent feedings, finger foods, frequent nutritional snacks).
3. Activity/exercise — potential need for restrictions based on cardiac status.	Assess current activity level. Determine what is tolerable activity based on cardiac status. Instruct child/parent in alternatives to activity level as diagnosis indicates. Evaluate need for frequency for naps or rest periods. Seek child's interests and help parent(s) establish routine for nap, active play, quiet play patterns.
4. Role relationship — potential alteration in socialization of child and parenting process due to chronic illness of a child.	Assess parent(s) need for counseling in dealing with altered social experiences of the young child. Discuss potential problems in the child's adaptation to chronic illness and altered ability to perform in the socialization process. Seek appropriate counseling as indicated with pediatric specialists.

5. Coping — stress tolerance due to reaction to child's anomaly.

Investigate ability of parent(s) to deal with diagnosis of child's anomaly as evidenced by their reaction to an interaction with child. Encourage child to express feelings regarding diagnosis and potential alterations in lifestyle (the teenage cardiac patient also must deal with the stress of developing during the adolescent years). Provide open, frank discussions about fears/concerns and plans for future lifestyle.

REFERRAL INFORMATION

Emotional/psychological development — include current growth/development information as well as reaction to diagnosis and potential lifestyle changes.

DRG 138

MDC 05	RW$ 0.9297	Medical	Outlier Cutoff 26	Mean LOS 5.7

Cardiac Arrhythmia and Conduction Disorders, Age > = 70 and/or CC

PRINCIPAL DIAGNOSIS WITH POTENTIAL HOME CARE NEEDS

Cardiac arrhythmia and conduction disorders

DETAILS TO CONSIDER

Patients dealing with long-term cardiac arrhythmia and/or conduction disorders have often experienced previous cardiac conditions that warranted surgical intervention. Long-term medical therapy may therefore be based on the need for drug therapy, pacemaker implantation, hypertension plus CHF follow-up and recurrent angina pectoris.

See Circulation **DRGs (103–107, 109, 115, 118, 121, 122, 124–127).**

POTENTIAL HOME CARE PROBLEMS

1. Potential nutritional habit alteration to maintain optimum performance of drug therapy.

2. Cognitive/perceptual pattern — knowledge deficit about disease process and potential complications from arrhythmia.

PLAN

Review dietary habits with patient to determine potential complications due to inappropriate diet coupled with specific medication therapy (diuretics, anticoagulants, etc.). Instruct patient in dietary restrictions as indicated.

Assess patient's understanding of drug therapy pertinent to condition to include dose, administration, expected actions, side effects and potential problems such as digitalis toxicity, bleeding from anticoagulation, hypotension, hypokalemia, etc. Instruct patient in monitoring of blood pressure as well as pulse and keeping record of results.

REFERRAL INFORMATION

Dependent on patient compliance and reaction to diagnosis.

| MDC 05 | RW$ 0.8303 | Medical | Outlier Cutoff 23 | Mean LOS 4.8 |

Cardiac Arrhythmia and Conduction Disorders
Age < 70 w/o CC

See **DRG 138**.

| MDC 05 | RW$ 0.7548 | Medical | Outlier Cutoff 21 | Mean LOS 5.5 |

Angina Pectoris

PRINCIPAL DIAGNOSIS WITH POTENTIAL HOME CARE NEEDS

Angina pectoris

DETAILS TO CONSIDER

Patients dealing with angina pectoris have had a long-standing history of coronary disease which has led to ischemic changes in the heart muscle. The range in severity can reach from *stable* (unchanged for several months) to *intractable*. Therapy is aimed at reducing myocardial oxygen demand and increasing oxygen supply. Treatment can range from rest and medication to coronary artery bypass.

See Circulatory **DRGs (121, 124–126, 132** and **134)**.

POTENTIAL HOME CARE PROBLEMS

PLAN

1. Cognitive/perceptual pattern — knowledge deficit regarding disease process.

See **DRG 132**.
Instruct patient in evaluation and management of chest pain to include ability to describe type of pain, quality, duration, severity, timing and likely precipitating factors. Use prescribed medications including dosage, expected effects, side effects and precautions in use with other medications and routine for resting activity along with potential for extension of disease process which may require coronary surgery.

2. Self-perception/self-concept — potential for depression.

Encourage verbalization about anxieties and fears. Investigate current work situation (is angina under control so that patient can resume previous work? if not, what are the alternatives for patient?) Has patient's role in the family been altered due to disease process and increased dependency? How will patient deal with role changes?

REFERRAL INFORMATION

Dependent upon extent of disability with disease process.

DRG 141

MDC 05	RW$ 0.6475	Medical	Outlier Cutoff 21	Mean LOS 5.0

Syncope and Collapse – Age > = 70 and/or CC

PRINCIPAL DIAGNOSES WITH POTENTIAL HOME CARE NEEDS

Orthostatic hypotension
Syncope and collapse

DETAILS TO CONSIDER

Syncope is often an indication of a critical reduction in cardiac output which leads to cerebral ischemia. Causes of such a reduction in output may include arrhythmias, a type of heart block, carotid sinus sensitivity or cerebrovascular obstructive disease. Treatment is dependent upon underlying disease process.

Orthostatic hypotension, as its name implies, is usually a transient disease in blood pressure due to sudden positional changes which result in reduction of circulation to the brain. Again, treatment is dependent upon causative agent.

POTENTIAL HOME CARE PROBLEM	PLAN
Potential for injury	Teaching of safety precautions is based on underlying disease process causing syncope events (see DRG specific to underlying disease). Review precautions in all activity levels required based on diagnosis/prognosis.

DRG 142

MDC 05	RW$ 0.5680	Medical	Outlier Cutoff 18	Mean LOS 4.3

Syncope and Collapse – Age < 70 w/o CC

PRINCIPAL DIAGNOSES WITH POTENTIAL HOME CARE NEEDS

Orthostatic hypotension
Syncope and collapse

See **DRG 141.**

| MDC 05 | RW$ 0.6814 | Medical | Outlier Cutoff 19 | Mean LOS 4.4 |

Chest Pain

PRINCIPAL DIAGNOSES WITH POTENTIAL HOME CARE NEEDS

Chest pain not otherwise specified.
Precordial pain

DETAILS TO CONSIDER

Precordial pain is often associated with positive identification of a precordial rub; in cases of pericarditis this condition often appears secondary to inflammation post-cardiac surgery and may be due to bacterial infections. Treatment is based on positive identification of pericarditis with antibiotic and steroid therapy. Potential home care problems are based on underlying cause of pericarditis.

See specific **DRGs.**

| MDC 05 | RW$ 1.1267 | Medical | Outlier Cutoff 27 | Mean LOS 7.0 |

Other Circulatory Diagnoses with CC

PRINCIPAL DIAGNOSES WITH POTENTIAL HOME CARE NEEDS

Myocardial degeneration
Heart injury
Neoplasm of heart

DETAILS TO CONSIDER

Myxomas (benign tumors originating from atrial septum) can cause obstruction to the mitral valve and present clinical picture of mitral stenosis. Surgical intervention is dependent upon the degree of stenosis (see specific DRG). Sarcomas (malignant tumors originating in the connective tissue of muscle walls) are usually identified after they have invaded the walls of the heart, causing obstruction in the blood supply and/or interrupting the normal contractivity of the heart. Death usually results from CHF or cardiac arrhythmias. Metastatic tumors from the breast, bronchus or lymph nodes often lead to pericardial effusion and constriction or obstruction of blood flow. Treatment is dependent upon underlying causes and potential for surgical intervention (see DRGs specific to surgical intervention). Inoperable situations are treated with supportive measures specific to complications (see specific DRGs related to treatment of CHF and cardiac arrythmias).

DRG 145

Other Circulatory Diagnoses w/o CC

See **DRG 144.**

6 MDC 06
DISEASES AND DISORDERS OF THE DIGESTIVE SYSTEM

Surgical Groupings (26 DRGs)

Rectal Resections

Major Small and Large Bowel Procedures

Minor Small and Large Bowel Procedures

Peritoneal Adhesiolysis

Stomach, Esophageal, Duodenal Procedures

Anal Procedures

Herniae

Appendectomy

Oral Surgery

Medical Groupings (19 DRGs)

Digestive Malignancy

GI Hemorrhage

Peptic Ulcer

Inflammatory Bowel Disease

GI Obstruction

Esophagitis

Gastroenteritis

Dental, Oral Diseases

MASTER HOME CARE PLANNING GUIDE
FOR CONDITIONS OF THE DIGESTIVE SYSTEM

Pattern	Assessment Factors	Plan
1. Health management deficit	Assess age of patient and age of caregiver, availability of primary caregiver for single person households. Assess financial status of patient and impact of long-term illness on family.	Interview primary caregiver and schedule visit to coincide with treatment caregiver will be required to do. Refer to social services for counseling.
2. Alteration in nutrition	Emphasis on nutritional status is indicated because almost any condition of the GI system interrupts the nutritional pattern.	See specific DRG.
3. Alteration in elimination	Emphasis on bowel elimination is also indicated. Some GI system conditions result in diversion of the bowel, thus affecting bowel elimination.	See specific DRG.
4. Activity and exercise	Assess level of home management deficit as mild, moderate, severe, potential or chronic.	
4a. Home maintenance management deficit		Interview patient and family to determine living arrangements (especially toilet facilities), ability to procure supplies, transportation needs for follow-up care. If patient is elderly and has other illnesses, assess need for energy saving and safety equipment. Determine potential home management deficit taking into consideration: • diagnosis and prognosis. • level of self-care needed. • ability and availability of caregiver. If deficit is mild, evaluate need for referral. For moderate deficit, do a referral to a home care agency for a home evaluation. For severe deficit make a definite referral.
5. Cognitive perceptual deficit		
5a. Knowledge deficit related to self-care	Assess patient's ability to follow routine of self-care, knowledge of signs and symptoms of complications. Ability to follow instructions in diet self-care needs to be assessed.	Give patient instructions in writing regarding care and diet. Communicate to visiting nurse the level of self-care the patient has reached. See DRG for specific self-care needs.
5b. Pain management	Assess patient's pain threshold and plan for pain control through	Review comfort measures for pain relief with patient and

comfort measures, diversional activities. Try to teach patient to control pain without narcotics as some narcotics may affect the GI system as well as the patient's ability to do self-care and function within the family. Patients with conditions of the GI system that are long-term need counseling in pain control measures.

family member, i.e. back rubs, relaxation, heat application (check with physician), diet control (to prevent flatulence and cramping). Refer for friendly visitor and volunteer for diversion therapy.

6. Sleep-rest pattern deficit

Some patients with GI disease will need to use protective bed coverings or sleep in modified positions.

Instruct patient with self-care needs to schedule care to allow for sleep and rest. See specific DRG.

7. Self-perception or self-concept change

Patients with ostomies will need a great deal of support in adapting to change in self-image. Factors such as temporary or permanent ostomy and continent or continuous drainage ostomy should be taken into consideration. Surgery in the mouth area may also lead to self-image problems.

Refer to social services for counseling for patients with a major change in body image. Communicate patient's status to home care nurse.

8. Role-relationship disturbance

The patient with an ostomy or major surgery to the mouth may feel the need to become socially isolated. Assisting patient in self-care routine that will allow the patient to socialize is essential. Patients who will be returning to work must be counseled regarding self-care. For patients who cannot assume total self-care and will need a spouse, child or other RP to assist with care, there may be a role reversal and thus a drastic effect on the relationship.

Same as #7. Include family in counseling when the patient's illness will have the potential for family disruption.

9. Sexuality — reproductive pattern interference

Some bowel surgeries will have an impact on patient's ability to participate sexually. It is imperative that when this effect is a possibility, it be discussed with the physician and patient prior to discharge. No matter what the age of the patient, this issue needs to be addressed.

Discuss potential for sexual dysfunction with physician. Determine patient, spouse or RP neeed for counseling.

10. Coping tolerance

The prognosis of the patient cannot always be determined. Assessment of the patient's and family's ability to cope with the stress must be made. Diseases of the GI system may interrupt family meal patterns, socialization patterns and role patterns, and may be of a long-term nature. Coping is essential for compliance with medical regime.

Communicate to the home care nurse the patient's level of coping role patterns and potential for inadequate coping.

11. Value belief pattern distress

When there is a malignancy or a change in body image there may be a spiritual crisis.

Allow patient to verbalize and follow up requests of patient or family for spiritual counseling.

DRG 146

MDC 06   **RW$ 2.7082**   **Surgical**   **Outlier Cutoff 39**   **Mean LOS 19.1**

Rectal Resection – Age > = 70 and/or CC

OPERATIVE PROCEDURES WITH POTENTIAL HOME CARE NEEDS

Abdominal-perineal resection
Anterior rectal resection with colostomy
Rectal resection

DETAILS TO CONSIDER

Age of patient > 70 or < 70 with comorbidity and/or complication(s). Comorbidity diagnosis which may increase long-term needs: Diabetes (**DRGs 294** and **295**); Circulatory System (**DRGs 128, 134, 139, 140**). Complication which will affect long-term need: wound infection with incomplete closure.

POTENTIAL HOME CARE PROBLEMS	PLAN
1. Lack of knowledge related to ostomy care at home.	Refer to home care nurse for home care. Communicate the following information to the nurse: the amount of bowel involved which affects the consistency of stool; the type of appliance and vendor; the plan for stool control (i.e. irrigations or colostomy pouch); the patient's level of self-care; impediments to self-care because of age or other disease.
2. Problems related to rectal and perineal wounds.	Assess need for dressings and sitz bath. Describe type available for male and female patients. Teach patient: signs and symptoms of complications such as infection; serous drainage expected until wound is healed.
3. Altered nutritional status secondary to bowel surgery and/or age.	Diet plans aimed at stool and flatulence control should be reviewed prior to discharge. Include patient's level of understanding of diet. Assess patient's nutritional needs after discharge, such as ability to shop, need for meals-on-wheels. Evaluate potential electrolyte loss and vitamin loss which can occur from diarrhea or high fluid loss through the ostomy.
4. Impaired mobility secondary to muscle weakness and/or progression of disease.	Assess ambulation safety, ability to climb stairs if applicable. Refer to physical therapy for instruction in energy saving and safety during ambulation. Assess ability of caregiver to assist in ambulation. Assess need for home health aide. Assess need for commode if patient will be confined to his/her bedroom for a period of time.

132

5. Alteration in body image, sexuality and family relationships.

Determine from physician the expected impact of surgery on sexual function. If patient will be unable to function sexually, discuss alternatives with patient. Communicate this to the home care nurse *regardless of the age of the patient,* for follow-up counseling. In patients who will need a spouse, child or other RP to assist with care, evaluate the effect of this on the family unit. There may be role reversal and thus the need for the home care nurse to counsel the caregiver.

6. Need for follow-up care.

Assess the transportation needs of the patient for follow-up care and the patient's understanding of its importance.

7. Durable medical equipment needs.

Sitz bath for perineal wound care. Bedside commode for patients who are confined to their room. Walker for impaired ambulation. Bathtub seat and hand rails may be needed.

REFERRAL INFORMATION

Background information — communicate pertinent health history of patient including comorbidity status and pertinent family history and living arrangements with regard to bedroom, bathroom, stairs and food preparation facilities. Current hospitalization history including complications — type of surgery and type of colostomy. Name of enterostomal therapist involved. Patient's understanding of the disease with regard to stool control, diet, care of the ostomy and perineal wound. Patient's ability to ambulate whether independently, with supervision or with a walker.

Plans for home care — description and availability of potential caregiver such as spouse, child, other RP. Potential need for home health aide. Relationship of patient to family members, especially spouse, in regard to sexual function. Durable medical equipment — what was ordered, from whom and length of time anticipated that the specific equipment will be needed.

DRG 147

MDC 06 **RW$ 2.5087** **Surgical** **Outlier Cutoff 38** **Mean LOS 17.9**

Rectal Resection – Age < 70 w/o CC

OPERATIVE PROCEDURES WITH POTENTIAL HOME CARE NEEDS

Abdominal perineal resection
Anterior rectal resection with colostomy

DETAILS TO CONSIDER

Patient is less than 70. Patient has no comorbidity or complication.

POTENTIAL HOME CARE PROBLEMS	PLAN
1. Lack of knowledge related to ostomy care at home.	Assess patient's level of understanding and ability to do self-care. Give patient instructions *in writing* regarding schedule of bowel care, type of equipment needed and where to buy it. Give detailed instructions on ostomy care. If available, refer patient to ostomy (enterostomal therapy) nurse for complete instruction.
2. Problems related to perineal wound.	Assess patient's need for a portable sitz bath or ability to use bathtub. Teach patient signs and symptoms of infection and that serous drainage is expected until wound is healed. Describe choices of wound dressing for male and female patients. Be aware of patient's needs for clothing protection if patient will be returning to usual activities before wound is completely healed.
3. Altered nutritional status secondary to surgery.	Do diet teaching or refer to dietician so patient can avoid stool problems related to diet, such as diarrhea, flatulence or constipation.
4. Alteration in body image, sexuality and family relationships.	Determine patient's lifestyle, plans to return to work and/or athletic pursuits. Refer to medical social worker or sex therapist for counseling in possible changes in lifestyle. The most important function of the nurse is to make the patient aware of sources of help available in follow-up care.

REFERRAL INFORMATION

Determine individual's need for the following: home care nurse; United Ostomy Association; medical social worker; sex therapist; enterostomal therapist; dietician; ostomy supply source.

| MDC 06 | RW$ 2.5493 | Surgical | Outlier Cutoff 37 | Mean LOS 17.0 |

Major Small and Large Bowel Procedures
Age >= 70 and/or CC

OPERATIVE PROCEDURES WITH POTENTIAL HOME CARE NEEDS

Perineal fistulae/various sites
Ileostomy/including temporary
Bowel anastomoses
Colostomy

DETAILS TO CONSIDER

Age of patient > 70 or < 70 with comorbidity and/or complication. Comorbidity which may increase home care needs: Diabetes (**DRGs 294, 295**); Circulatory System (**DRGs 128, 134, 138, 140**). Complication which will affect long-term care: Infection (**DRG 149**). Fistulae formation may be a chronic condition. Length of time for a temporary ostomy may not be determined; therefore length of time for home care is indefinite.

POTENTIAL HOME CARE PROBLEMS	PLAN
See **Master Care Plan** for MDC 06, and see **DRGs 146** and **147**.	
1. Alteration in nutrition.	Potential for trauma from diet, fluid and electrolyte imbalance exists. Get a specific diet order from the physician. Consider other health problems such as diabetic diet or low sodium diet.
2. Alteration in elimination.	The plan for bowel evacuation must be specific. In some types of surgery in this DRG, constipation to rest the rectum is desired; in others, soft stool formation is desired.

| MDC 06 | RW$ 2.2154 | Surgical | Outlier Cutoff 35 | Mean LOS 15.2 |

Major Small and Large Bowel Procedures – Age < 70 w/o CC

OPERATIVE PROCEDURES WITH POTENTIAL HOME CARE NEEDS

Perineal fistulae/various sites
Ileostomy/including temporary
Bowel anastomosis
Colostomy

DETAILS TO CONSIDER

Patient is less than 70. Length of time patient will have temporary ostomy is indefinite at the time of discharge. Perineal fistulae may be a chronic condition. Refer to **DRG 138**.

DRG 150

MDC 06   **RW$ 2.3746**   **Surgical**   **Outlier Cutoff 35**   **Mean LOS 15.3**

Peritoneal Adhesiolysis – Age > = 70 and/or CC

OPERATIVE PROCEDURES WITH POTENTIAL HOME CARE NEEDS

Perineal fistulae/various sites
Ileostomy/including temporary
Bowel anastomosis
Colostomy

DETAILS TO CONSIDER

Adhesions are abnormal attachments between peritoneal surfaces. Most are inflammatory in origin and follow either a surgical operation or peritonitis. The chief complication is intestinal obstruction. The patient is > 70. Comorbidity which may increase long-term needs: other abdominal surgery or recent peritonitis will result in a compromised patient. Complications which will affect long-term illness: incomplete wound closure; nutritional depletions.

POTENTIAL HOME CARE PROBLEMS

1. Alteration in nutrition.

2. Self-care needs.

PLAN

Assess need for long-term nutritional supplement. Diet orders must take into consideration patient's preexisting problem.

Evaluate existing health care needs and reinforce previous teaching and health care routine. If patient was receiving health care services prior to admission, reinstitute services, including new information. Refer to dietician for assessment, diet planning and diet teaching, especially if other diseases exist such as diabetes or heart disease.

Peritoneal Adhesiolysis – Age < 70 w/o CC

OPERATIVE PROCEDURES WITH POTENTIAL HOME CARE NEEDS

Same as **DRG 150.**

DETAILS TO CONSIDER

Adhesions are abnormal attachments between peritoneal surfaces. Most are inflammatory in origin and follow surgery on peritonitis. Recurrence of adhesions in patients with a predisposition to adhesions is possible.

Refer to **DRG 150.**

POTENTIAL HOME CARE PROBLEMS

See **Master Care Plan** for MDC 06.

PLAN

1. Alteration in nutrition.

Assess need for long-term nutritional supplement. Diet orders must take into consideration preexisting condition. Evaluate patient's need for nutritional supplement.

2. Self-care needs.

Evaluate existing health care needs. Reinforce previous teaching and health care routine.

REFERRAL INFORMATION

If patient was receiving health care services prior to admission, reinstate services.

Minor Small and Large Bowel Procedures > = 70 and/or CC

OPERATIVE PROCEDURES WITH POTENTIAL HOME CARE NEEDS

Stoma closure/small and large bowel

DETAILS TO CONSIDER

Unless patient has significant comorbidity, home care is not indicated. Predischarge teaching regarding diet and follow-up care is essential.

REFERRAL INFORMATION

If patient was receiving home care primarily because of other health problems, refer back to the home care agency for evaluation.

DRG 153

MDC 06	RW$ 1.2599	Surgical	Outlier Cutoff 29	Mean LOS 9.3

Minor Small and Large Bowel Procedures – Age < 70 w/o CC

OPERATIVE PROCEDURES WITH POTENTIAL HOME CARE NEEDS

Stoma closure/small and large bowel

DETAILS TO CONSIDER

When discharged, patient should be independent in care. Level of care will be less intense. Home care is not indicated. Refer to **DRG 152.**

DRG 154

MDC 06	RW$ 2.6901	Surgical	Outlier Cutoff 35	Mean LOS 14.8

Stomach, Esophageal and Duodenal Procedures Age > = 70 and/or CC

OPERATIVE PROCEDURES WITH POTENTIAL HOME CARE NEEDS

Esophagectomy with anastomosis
Injection and ligation of esophageal varices
Gastrectomy/total and partial
Diaphragmatic hernia

DETAILS TO CONSIDER

Patients in this DRG have different needs depending on anatomical location and reason for surgery. The patient with (1) esophageal surgery, (2) gastric surgery and (3) diaphragmatic hernia will be treated separately. Therefore three different plans are to be considered. Comorbidity affecting long-term needs includes obesity and alcoholism.

Refer to **DRGs 155, 173** and **182.**

Esophageal Surgery

POTENTIAL HOME CARE PROBLEMS	PLAN
1. Alteration in nutrition.	Determine potential for patient to swallow food. Determine mechanism by which the patient will receive nutrients (example; by nasogastric tube, gastrostomy tube, jejunostomy tube or parenterally — or if he/she will be able to eat a modified diet. Get a specific diet order from the physician including mechanical characteristics and fat content of the diet.

2. Alteration in elimination.

Inform patient that bowel pattern may change depending on source of nutrition.

3. Self-care needs.

After determining long-term plan, instruct patient in care of tube, either nasogastric or other. Give patient instructions in writing.

4. Sleep, rest patterns.

Patient should sleep in upright position if on tube feedings. Evaluate need for hospital bed at home to facilitate positioning.

5. Durable medical equipment needs.

Hospital bed. Enteral feeding pump.

REFERRAL INFORMATION

Refer to visiting nurse for: tube feeding regime, understanding of enteral feeding pump if applicable; monitoring of elimination pattern depending on source of nutrition; care of tube insertion site and tube patency. If patient has esophageal varices, be aware that other serious abdominal problems probably also exist. Chronic hepatitis and alcohol abuse may exist. Alcohol abuse counseling may be indicated.

Gastric Surgery

POTENTIAL HOME CARE PROBLEMS

PLAN

1. Alteration in nutrition.

Get a specific diet order from the physician. Take into account that nutritional impairment frequently occurs after gastric surgery. Refer to dietician for individualized diet teaching. Assess for potential of "dumping syndrome".

2. Alteration in elimination.

Inform patient that bowel pattern may change depending on type of surgery and type of diet.

3. Sleep, rest position.

If "dumping syndrome" is expected, instruct patient to lie down after eating to delay emptying of the stomach. Be careful when giving this advice because of potential for regurgitation with resultant aspiration, pneumonia and esophageal irritation.

REFERRAL INFORMATION

These patients should not need referral unless other diseases exist.

Diaphragmatic Hernia

POTENTIAL HOME CARE PROBLEMS

PLAN

1. Alteration in nutrition.

Instruct patient to eat small, frequent meals and avoid spiced foods.

2. Alteration in elimination.

Instruct patient to avoid straining during bowel evacuation. Patient may need stool softener.

3. Sleep, rest pattern.

Instruct patient to remain in sitting position 1–2 hours after eating.

REFERRAL INFORMATION

Unless other diseases exist, no referral should be needed.

DRG 155

MDC 06	RW$ 2.3336	Surgical	Outlier Cutoff 33	Mean LOS 13.0

Stomach, Esophageal and Duodenal Procedures
Age 18–69 w/o CC

OPERATIVE PROCEDURES WITH POTENTIAL HOME CARE NEEDS

Esophagectomy with anastomosis
Injection and ligation of esophageal varices
Gastrectomy/total and partial
Gastric surgeries
Diaphragmatic hernia

See **DRG 154** and **DRG 182.**

DRG 156

MDC 06	RW$ 0.8470	Surgical	Outlier Cutoff 20	Mean LOS 6.0

Stomach, Esophageal and Duodenal Procedures – Age 0–17

OPERATIVE PROCEDURES WITH POTENTIAL HOME CARE NEEDS

Esophageal surgeries
Gastric surgeries

DETAILS TO CONSIDER

Because of age of patient, posthospital care will be done by parent or other RP. Review **DRG 154** and include parent or other RP in all teaching sessions.

REFERRAL INFORMATION

Refer to a home care nurse if child is very young. Parent will need guidance in care of condition and in understanding developmental needs of the patient. Family may need social service referral if illness has potential to cause coping problems.

| MDC 06 | RW$ 0.7985 | Surgical | Outlier Cutoff 25 | Mean LOS 6.0 |

Anal Procedures – Age > = 70 and/or CC

OPERATIVE PROCEDURES WITH POTENTIAL HOME CARE NEEDS

Stoma revision
Perianal fistulae and abscess
Hemorrhoidectomy/cryotherapy/ligation
Pericolostomy hernia repair

DETAILS TO CONSIDER

Procedures in this category are relatively minor with a relatively short LOS.

Refer to **Master Care Plan MDC 06.**

POTENTIAL HOME CARE PROBLEMS

PLAN

1. Alteration in nutrition.

Get specific diet order from physician when protection of anal wound is indicated. Take into consideration other health problems.

2. Alteration in elimination.

Determine needs as discussed above. Determine need for stool softeners.

3. Self-care needs.

Determine need for revision in stoma care resulting from either revision or hernia. Teach patient how to care for anal wound, including hygiene measures.

REFERRAL INFORMATION

If patient was receiving home care prior to surgery, assess need for continuation of services.

Refer patient with stoma to enterostomal therapist for follow-up care. Size of stoma appliances may need to be changed for a short time after surgery to protect the patient's skin and stoma integrity.

| MDC 06 | RW$ 0.6408 | Surgical | Outlier Cutoff 19 | Mean LOS 5.2 |

Anal Procedures – Age < 70 w/o CC

OPERATIVE PROCEDURES WITH POTENTIAL HOME CARE NEEDS

Stoma revision
Perianal fistulae and abscess
Hemorrhoidectomy/cryotherapy/ligation
Pericolostomy hernia repair

Refer to **DRG 157.**

DRG 159

| MDC 06 | RW$ 0.9297 | Surgical | Outlier Cutoff 23 | Mean LOS 7.1 |

Hernia Procedures Except Inguinal and Femoral
Age > = 70 and/or CC

OPERATIVE PROCEDURES WITH POTENTIAL HOME CARE NEEDS

Umbilical herniorrhaphy
Incisional herniorrhaphy with graft

DETAILS TO CONSIDER

Comorbidity which may increase home care needs: obesity. Complication which may increase home care needs: incomplete wound closure.

POTENTIAL HOME CARE PROBLEMS

1. Alteration in nutrition.

2. Self-care deficit related to incomplete wound closure.

PLAN

If patient is obese and this has contributed to herniation, encourage dieting for weight reduction.

Assess patient's ability to do wound care, taking into consideration other health conditions. Patient should be able to do wound care if procedure is relatively easy.

REFERRAL INFORMATION

If patient was receiving home care prior to surgery because of other health problems, assess need for continuation of services. No new services should be needed unless patient will need skilled nurse for wound care.

DRG 160

| MDC 06 | RW$ 0.7676 | Surgical | Outlier Cutoff 18 | Mean LOS 6.0 |

Hernia Procedures Except Inguinal and Femoral
Age 18–69 w/o CC

OPERATIVE PROCEDURES WITH POTENTIAL HOME CARE NEEDS

Umbilical hernia
Incisional hernia with graft

See **DRG 159.**

MDC 06   RW$ 0.7068   Surgical   Outlier Cutoff 16   Mean LOS 5.7

Inguinal and Femoral Hernia Procedures
Age > = 70 and/or CC

OPERATIVE PROCEDURES WITH POTENTIAL HOME CARE NEEDS

Inguinal and femoral herniae

DETAILS TO CONSIDER

A complication which may affect home care needs is incomplete wound closure. Involvement of male reproductive system may occur in some hernia repair. Hernia repair may be done through peritoneal incisions.

See **DRG 159.**

POTENTIAL HOME CARE PROBLEM

Sexual dysfunction secondary to surgical intervention.

PLAN

Determine from physician the potential effect on sexual function in the male patient. Communicate information to the patient. Even if there is *no* interruption or no anticipated interruption, communicate this to the patient.

REFERRAL INFORMATION

Conditions in this DRG normally do not have home care needs. Many are done in day surgery settings.

MDC 06   RW$ 0.5854   Surgical   Outlier Cutoff 12   Mean LOS 4.8

Inguinal and Femoral Hernia Procedures
Age 18–69 w/o CC

OPERATIVE PROCEDURES WITH POTENTIAL HOME CARE NEEDS

Same as **DRG 161.**

DRG 163

MDC 06	RW$ 0.4358	Surgical	Outlier Cutoff 6	Mean LOS 2.1

Hernia Procedures – Age 0–17

OPERATIVE PROCEDURES WITH POTENTIAL HOME CARE NEEDS

Umbilical
Incisional
Femoral
Inguinal
Repair of gastroschisis

DETAILS TO CONSIDER

Patients with hernia in this age group do not usually have home care needs. A gastroschisis is a full-thickness abdominal wall defect which is treated with surgery at birth. There may also be other related anomalies.

POTENTIAL HOME CARE PROBLEM	PLAN
Alteration in parenting.	Parents may need follow-up counseling in dealing with child whose anomaly is visible and alarming at birth. Child may also have other anomalies causing concern.

REFERRAL INFORMATION

The reader is referred to pediatric texts for additional information.

DRG 164

MDC 06	RW$ 1.8320	Surgical	Outlier Cutoff 32	Mean LOS 11.9

Appendectomy with Complicated Principal Diagnosis
Age > = 70 and/or CC

Complicated principal diagnosis: malignant neoplasm of appendix; acute appendix with peritonitis; abscess of appendix

OPERATIVE PROCEDURES WITH POTENTIAL HOME CARE NEEDS

Appendectomy
Drain appendiceal abscess

DETAILS TO CONSIDER

Patient may have additional comorbidity such as diabetes or heart disease. The patient may be acutely ill on admission and may be unstable because the symptoms of appendicitis in the elderly are often vague and do not localize until later. In most cases where there is peritonitis or abscess, a drain is usually in place to allow for escape of purulent material.

See **Master Care Plan MDC 06.**

POTENTIAL HOME CARE PROBLEMS

1. Self-care deficit related to draining and open surgical wound.

2. Sleep, rest pattern.

3. Durable medical equipment needs.

PLAN

Determine estimate of time before there will be wound closure. Following specific physician's orders for posthospital wound care, teach patient how to do wound care if possible. If not, refer to visiting nurse for wound care and assessment of other home care needs. Be sure plans for care include maintaining skin integrity around the wound.

Maintaining semi-Fowler's position facilitates wound drainage and decreases chance for spread of infection.

Evaluate for need of hospital bed to facilitate semi-Fowler's position to drain abscess.

REFERRAL INFORMATION

Refer to a home care nurse for wound care in the home. Communicate doctor's orders for wound care, supplies needed, technique used and patient's level of self-care.

Refer also for evaluation of need for home health aide if patient was acutely ill prior to surgery.

DRG 165

MDC 06	RW$ 1.6154	Surgical	Outlier Cutoff 29	Mean LOS 11.3

Appendectomy with Complicated Principal Diagnosis Age < 70 w/o CC

Complicated principal diagnosis: malignant neoplasm of appendix; acute appendix with peritonitis; abscess of appendix

OPERATIVE PROCEDURES WITH POTENTIAL HOME CARE NEEDS

Appendectomy
Drain appendiceal abscess

See **DRG 164.**

DRG 166

MDC 06	RW$ 1.4328	Surgical	Outlier Cutoff 29	Mean LOS 9.4

Appendectomy w/o Complicated Principal Diagnosis Age > = 70 and/or CC

OPERATIVE PROCEDURES WITH POTENTIAL HOME CARE NEEDS

Appendectomy
Drain appendiceal abscess

See **DRG 164.**

DRG 167

MDC 06	RW$ 1.0818	Surgical	Outlier Cutoff 22	Mean LOS 7.4

Appendectomy w/o Complicated Principal Diagnosis Age < 70 w/o CC

OPERATIVE PROCEDURES WITH POTENTIAL HOME CARE NEEDS

Appendectomy
Drain appendiceal abscess

See **DRG 164.**

MDC 06　　**RW$ 0.8631**　　**Surgical**　　**Outlier Cutoff 24**　　**Mean LOS 4.3**

Procedures on the Mouth – Age > = 70 and/or CC

OPERATIVE PROCEDURES WITH POTENTIAL HOME CARE NEEDS

Plastic repair of palate
Radical neck dissection
Total mandibulectomy with reconstruction
Other osteoplasty of facial bones

DETAILS TO CONSIDER

Operative procedures of the mouth affect the GI system and have a direct effect on the respiratory system. Comorbidity which will affect long-term needs: lung diseases (see **MDC 04**).

POTENTIAL HOME CARE PROBLEMS	PLAN
1. Alteration in nutrition related to oral procedure.	Assess patient's ability to eat. Patient may need liquid diet or feeding tube to bypass surgical site. If patient has feeding tube, determine patient's ability to self-feed.
2. Potential alteration in respiratory status.	If patient has respiratory disease with a productive cough, assess the need for suction to help patient keep the airway clear. Assess the need for continuous oxygen in the home.
3. Self-care needs.	Determine wound care and suction needs. Also determine the best method for oral hygiene, including irrigation.
4. Durable medical equipment needs.	Portable suction machine. Potential need for oxygen.

REFERRAL INFORMATION

Refer to home care nurse for wound care, oral irrigations and evaluation of patient's ability to self-suction. If wounds are a result of trauma, refer to social service worker for counseling.

DRG 169

MDC 06   **RW$ 0.8992**   **Surgical**   **Outlier Cutoff 24**   **Mean LOS 4.2**

Procedures on the Mouth – Age < 70 w/o CC

OPERATIVE PROCEDURES WITH POTENTIAL HOME CARE NEEDS

Plastic repair of palate
Radical neck dissection
Total mandibulectomy with reconstruction
Other osteoplasty of facial bones

DETAILS TO CONSIDER

See **DRG 168.**

DRG 170

MDC 06   **RW$ 2.6602**   **Surgical**   **Outlier Cutoff 35**   **Mean LOS 14.6**

Other Digestive System Procedures – Age > = 70 and/or CC

DETAILS TO CONSIDER

Diagnoses in this group are grouped because of similarity in resource consumption. conditions with potential for home care needs are covered elsewhere under specific systems.

DRG 171

MDC 06   **RW$ 2.3976**   **Surgical**   **Outlier Cutoff 33**   **Mean LOS 13.3**

Other Digestive System Procedures – Age < 70 w/o CC

See **DRG 170.**

| MDC 06 | RW$ 1.2268 | Medical | Outlier Cutoff 28 | Mean LOS 8.2 |

Digestive Malignancy – Age > = 70 and/or CC

PRINCIPAL DIAGNOSES WITH POTENTIAL HOME CARE NEEDS

Malignant neoplasm of: esophagus; stomach; pylorus; small intestine (duodenum, jejunum, ileum); colon; appendix; rectum; anus; peritoneum

Refer to **DRG 146** (rectal), **DRG 148** (bowel), **DRG 154** (stomach, esophagus, duodenum), **DRG 168** (mouth).

DETAILS TO CONSIDER

The plan for home care will depend on several factors including the following: (1) stage of disease, (2) type of treatment, such as chemotherapy and/or radiation, (3) prognosis, (4) family support system.

The patient may have had prior surgery for neoplasm and is now being treated medically.

POTENTIAL HOME CARE PROBLEMS

Refer to **Master Care Plan MDC 06.**

PLAN

POTENTIAL HOME CARE PROBLEMS	PLAN
1. Alteration in nutrition.	Assess patient's nutritional needs and ability to eat. Get a specific diet order and give the diet instructions to the patient in writing. Refer to dietician or oncology clinician for specific nutrition problems.
2. Home maintenance management impairment.	Taking above factors into consideration, evaluate patient and family's ability to manage patient at home.

REFERRAL INFORMATION

Refer to a home care nurse for monitoring of effects of therapy and progression of disease. If patient is terminal, refer for hospice service.

| MDC 06 | RW$ 1.0517 | Medical | Outlier Cutoff 27 | Mean LOS 6.7 |

Digestive Malignancy – Age < 70 w/o CC

See **DRG 172.**

DRG 174

MDC 06	RW$ 0.9281	Medical	Outlier Cutoff 27	Mean LOS 6.7

GI Hemorrhage – Age > = 70 and/or CC

PRINCIPAL DIAGNOSES WITH POTENTIAL HOME CARE NEEDS

Principal diagnosis: esophageal varices with bleeding; stomach ulcers with bleeding; duodenal ulcers; peptic ulcers with bleeding; rectal/anal hemorrhage; hematemesis/melena;

Refer to **DRG 146** (rectal), **DRG 148** (bowel), **DRG 154** (stomach, esophagus, duodenum), **DRG 168** (mouth).

DETAILS TO CONSIDER

GI hemorrhage is a symptom of disease. The plan of treatment must be directed at the disease process and not the symptom. When the site of bleeding is determined, the plan of care can be made. Surgical intervention may be indicated depending on the severity of bleeding.

DRG 175

MDC 06	RW$ 0.8236	Medical	Outlier Cutoff 24	Mean LOS 5.8

GI Hemorrhage – Age < 70 w/o CC

See **DRG 174**.

MDC 06   **RW$ 1.2438**   **Medical**   **Outlier Cutoff 28**   **Mean LOS 8.1**

Complicated Peptic Ulcer

PRINCIPAL DIAGNOSES WITH POTENTIAL HOME CARE NEEDS

GI tract ulceration with obstruction or perforation
Meckel's diverticulum (of ileum)
Acquired pyloric stenosis

DETAILS TO CONSIDER

No age differentiation for complicated peptic ulcer. Peptic ulcers are an erosion of the lining of the stomach or duodenum. The acquired pyloric stenosis results from the caustic action of gastric acid with resultant scarring near the pylorus. Treatment for these complications may be surgical or dietary.

Refer to **DRG 154.**

POTENTIAL HOME CARE PROBLEM	PLAN
Alteration in nutrition.	Specific diet orders should be written by the physician. Diet which is relatively bland chemically, thermally and mechanically. Modification of eating pattern may need to be reinforced.

DRG 177

MDC 06   **RW$ 0.7422**   **Medical**   **Outlier Cutoff 24**   **Mean LOS 6.6**

Uncomplicated Peptic Ulcer – Age > = 70 and/or CC

PRINCIPAL DIAGNOSES WITH POTENTIAL HOME CARE NEEDS

Stomach ulcers
Duodenal ulcers
Peptic ulcers

DETAILS TO CONSIDER

This condition can be related to coping — stress tolerance pattern. It can be successfully treated with medication/diet regime. Long-term needs exist only where there is a comorbidity.

DRG 178

MDC 06 **RW$ 0.6141** **Medical** **Outlier Cutoff 20** **Mean LOS 5.5**

Uncomplicated Peptic Ulcer – Age < 70 w/o CC

PRINCIPAL DIAGNOSES WITH POTENTIAL HOME CARE NEEDS

Stomach ulcers
Duodenal ulcers
Peptic ulcers

See **DRG 177.**

DRG 179

MDC 06 **RW$ 1.0153** **Medical** **Outlier Cutoff 28** **Mean LOS 8.0**

Inflammatory Bowel Disease

PRINCIPAL DIAGNOSES WITH POTENTIAL HOME CARE NEEDS

Regional enteritis, small and large intestine
Idiopathic proctocolitis

DETAILS TO CONSIDER

No age differentiation, but it is a problem most frequently seen in young people.

POTENTIAL HOME CARE PROBLEMS	PLAN
1. Alteration in nutrition.	Obtain a specific diet order from the physician.
2. Alteration in elimination.	Frequent diarrheal stools may lead to fluid and electrolyte imbalances. Diarrhea, pain and cramping are treated symptomatically.
3. Self-perception disturbance.	This disease can have many effects on the socialization of the young adult. Investigate the need for counseling.

REFERRAL INFORMATION

Home care needs are minimal in most cases except where the patient has become debilitated.

If patient needs additional nutrition instruction or needs to be monitored for fluid and electrolyte balance refer to a home care nurse.

MDC 06   **RW$ 0.8197**   **Medical**   **Outlier Cutoff 26**   **Mean LOS 6.2**

GI Obstruction – Age > = 70 and/or CC

PRINCIPAL DIAGNOSES WITH POTENTIAL HOME CARE NEEDS

Intussusception
Paralytic ileus
Volvulus of intestine
Impaction of intestine
Intestinal obstruction

DETAILS TO CONSIDER

Obstruction of the small intestine can sometimes be safely treated using an intestinal tube to decompress the bowel. If the obstruction is only partial, the upper GI tract may regain some degree of function. Obstruction of the colon cannot usually be treated by decompression and chance of perforation is greater in the colon. Long-term needs will depend on the type of obstruction, the medical or surgical treatment and the cause.

Refer to **DRG 146** (bowel procedures) and **DRG 173** (digestive malignancy).

MDC 06   **RW$ 0.7845**   **Medical**   **Outlier Cutoff 26**   **Mean LOS 5.9**

GI Obstruction – Age < 70 w/o CC

PRINCIPAL DIAGNOSES WITH POTENTIAL HOME CARE NEEDS

Intussusception
Paralytic ileus
Volvulus of intestine
Impaction of intestine
Intestinal obstruction

See **DRG 180.**

DRG 182

MDC 06   **RW$ 0.6185**   **Medical**   **Outlier Cutoff 22**   **Mean LOS 5.4**

Esophagitis, Gastroenteritis and
Miscellaneous Digestive Disorders – Age > = 70 and/or CC

PRINCIPAL DIAGNOSES WITH POTENTIAL HOME CARE NEEDS

Various bacterial and viral enteritis; protozoan, parasitic or vermin infestations of the GI tract
Achalasia
Diaphragmatic hernia
Esophagitis, stricture and perforation
Acute gastritis
Alcoholic gastritis
Diverticulosis

DETAILS TO CONSIDER

Diagnoses in this group are grouped because they use similar resources. The conditions that result from infection or infestation of the GI tract have public health implications. Although the patient will have minimal home care needs, finding the source of illness is necessary; therefore reporting the illness to the Public Health Department is indicated.

Refer to **DRG 154** (esophagitis).

POTENTIAL HOME CARE PROBLEMS

PLAN

1. Alteration in nutrition.

Get a specific diet order from the physician. Take into consideration other diseases. Instruct the patient to eat small, frequent meals that are relatively bland chemically, thermally and mechanically. Avoid foods with seeds if diverticulosis is present.

2. Sleep, rest pattern.

Instruct patient to remain in semi-Fowler's position 1–2 hours after eating. If there is gastric regurgitation, encourage patient to sleep in semi-Fowler's position.

3. Durable equipment needs.

Assess need for hospital bed for maintenance of semi-Fowler's position.

REFERRAL INFORMATION

If patient had been receiving home care prior to hospitalization, evaluate for additional needs. In cases of GI infection or infestation, report illness to public health agency for follow-up on contacts. Assess need for substance abuse counseling.

| MDC 06 | RW$ 0.5652 | Medical | Outlier Cutoff 19 | Mean LOS 4.8 |

Esophagitis, Gastroenteritis and Miscellaneous Digestive Disorders – Age 18–69 w/o CC

PRINCIPAL DIAGNOSES WITH POTENTIAL HOME CARE NEEDS

Various bacterial and viral enteritis; protozoan, parasitic or vermin infestations of the GI tract.
Achalasia
Diaphragmatic hernia
Esophagitis, stricture and perforation
Acute gastritis
Alcoholic gastritis
Diverticulosis

See DRG 182.

| MDC 06 | RW$ 0.3822 | Medical | Outlier Cutoff 11 | Mean LOS 3.3 |

Esophagitis, Gastroenteritis and Miscellaneous Disorders – Age 0–17

PRINCIPAL DIAGNOSES WITH POTENTIAL HOME CARE NEEDS

Various bacterial and viral enteritis, protozoan, parasitic or vermin infestations
Esophageal perforation or other esophageal disorders
Gastritis
Celiac disease

DETAILS TO CONSIDER

See DRG 182.

Celiac disease can occur at any age but is most frequently found in young children.

POTENTIAL HOME CARE PROBLEM

Alteration in nutrition.

PLAN

Get specific diet order from physician. Do diet teaching with parent. Counsel adolescent patient in diet, allowing for variations as needed for socialization.

REFERRAL INFORMATION

Because LOS is short, refer to a home care nurse for follow-up teaching and evaluation of progression of disease.

The reader is referred to pediatric texts for additional information.

DRG 185

MDC 06 **RW$ 0.6681** **Medical** **Outlier Cutoff 24** **Mean LOS 4.2**

Dental and Oral Diseases
Excluding Extractions and Restorations – Age > = 18

PRINCIPAL DIAGNOSES WITH POTENTIAL HOME CARE NEEDS

Malignant neoplasm of the lip, gum or cheek mucosa
Periodontitis
Gingivitis, acute, chronic
Dentofacial anomaly
Tongue disorders
Congenital defects of the mouth
Open wounds of the mouth, lip and jaw
Fracture of facial bones
Herpetic gingivostomatitis
Hard tissue disease of the teeth
Jaw disease

See **DRG 168.**

DETAILS TO CONSIDER

Long-term needs will depend on the effect on the patient's ability to eat and communicate and potential risk for airway obstruction. If condition results from trauma, follow-up reporting and counseling is indicated. History of congenital or rheumatic heart disease should alert caregiver to risk of bacterial endocarditis secondary to tooth decay.

POTENTIAL HOME CARE PROBLEMS

1. Alteration in nutrition secondary to difficulty in eating.

2. Alteration in elimination secondary to diet restriction.

3. Alteration in self-image related to visibility of the condition.

4. Potential alteration in respiration secondary to airway obstruction.

PLAN

Assess patient's nutritional needs to meet growth and development requirements. Patient may need a mechanically soft diet.

Assess patient's use of laxatives and recommend products that can be taken in liquid form, such as Metamucil.

Assess patient's ability to socialize following treatment in relation to appearance. If the surgical procedure has caused a "disfiguring" defect, allow patient to verbalize feelings. If there is a tendency toward social isolation, have patient seek counseling.

Assess patient's ability to clear mucus from the airway and to remove material in the event of vomiting.

5. Oral hygiene needs.

Instruct patient in oral hygiene. Oral lavage with a power spray device may be used *after* consulting with the physician. Some spray devices may be contraindicated in soft tissue disease. Mouth irrigations with normal saline or a weak sodium bicarbonate may be used. Caution against using breath mints with sugar for long periods of time because they may contribute to tooth decay. Instruct patient to expect some drooling and to carry tissues at all times.

REFERRAL INFORMATION

If condition was the result of trauma, refer to social services for follow-up. If condition has resulted in speech impairment of a long-term nature, refer to speech therapist.

DRG 186

MDC 06	RW$ 0.4155	Medical	Outlier Cutoff 11	Mean LOS 2.9

Dental and Oral Diseases
Excluding Extractions and Restorations – Age 0–17

PRINCIPAL DIAGNOSIS WITH POTENTIAL HOME CARE NEEDS

See **DRGs 168** and **185**.

DETAILS TO CONSIDER

Congenital conditions of the mouth can lead to eating problems and poor weight gain in children. Some congenital problems can be treated surgically early while others must be delayed until the mouth structure develops.

POTENTIAL HOME CARE PROBLEMS

1. Alteration in parenting secondary to congenital defect which is visible.

2. Alteration in socialization in the adolescent.

3. Alteration in nutrition.

PLAN

Counsel parents and allow them to verbalize their feelings.

If the adolescent is having difficulty socializing because of the oral defect, refer to counseling.

Assess nutritional needs to adequately meet growth needs. Plan supplements to meet the dietary needs. Methods of feeding the infant must be devised and instructions on how to position the infant to prevent postparandial aspiration is important.

REFERRAL INFORMATION

If parents appear to be having difficulty in coping, refer for counseling. If the mouth defect appears to be from trauma, determine nature of trauma and follow-up if indicated.

The reader is referred to pediatric texts for additional information.

DRG 187

| MDC 06 | RW$ 0.3990 | Medical/Surgical | Outlier Cutoff 8 | Mean LOS 2.7 |

Dental Extractions and Restorations

PRINCIPAL DIAGNOSES WITH POTENTIAL HOME CARE NEEDS

Dental extractions
Restorations

DETAILS TO CONSIDER

History of congenital or rheumatic heart disease should alert caregiver to the risk of sub-acute bacterial endocarditis.

See **DRGs 185** and **186.**

DRG 188

| MDC 06 | RW$ 0.7444 | Medical | Outlier Cutoff 25 | Mean LOS 5.1 |

Other Digestive System Diagnoses – Age $>$ = 70 and/or CC

PRINCIPAL DIAGNOSES WITH POTENTIAL HOME CARE NEEDS

Intestinal TB
Benign neoplasms of the GI tract
Hemorrhoids
Peritonitis
Injury to abdominal organs
Foreign body removal
Burn of the GI tract
Attention to gastrostomy, ileostomy and colostomy (not surgical procedure)

DETAILS TO CONSIDER

The long-term needs for patients in this DRG are discussed under other sections in this chapter and in the **Master Care Plan** at the beginning of the chapter.

Since this is a Medical DRG the patient will not have a surgical procedure.

Some of the conditions in this DRG are of a chronic nature, and the patient may be hospitalized for exacerbations of illness aggravated by comorbidity.

| MDC 06 | RW$ 0.6576 | Medical | Outlier Cutoff 23 | Mean LOS 4.5 |

Other Digestive System Diagnoses – Age 18–69 w/o CC

PRINCIPAL DIAGNOSIS WITH POTENTIAL HOME CARE NEEDS

See **DRG 188.**

DETAILS TO CONSIDER

Compare with **DRGs 173, 175, 178, 179, 181** and **183.**

| MDC 06 | RW$ 0.3379 | Medical | Outlier Cutoff 8 | Mean LOS 2.1 |

Other Digestive System Diagnoses – Age 0–17

PRINCIPAL DIAGNOSES WITH POTENTIAL HOME CARE NEEDS

Inflammatory bowel disease
Congenital esophageal fistula or atresia
Gastric and intestinal anomalies
Hirschsprung's disease (congenital megacolon)

See **DRG 188.**

DETAILS TO CONSIDER

Compare with **DRGs 156, 184** and **186.**

The reader is referred to pediatric texts for additional information.

7

MDC 07
DISEASES AND DISORDERS OF THE
HEPATOBILIARY SYSTEM AND PANCREAS

SURGICAL GROUPINGS (11 DRGs)

Major Pancreas, Liver and Shunt Procedures

Biliary Tract Procedures

Total Cholecystectomy

Hepatobiliary Diagnostic Procedures

Other Hepatobiliary and Pancreas OR Procedures

MEDICAL GROUPINGS (7 DRGs)

Cirrhosis and Alcoholic Hepatitis

Malignancy of Hepatobiliary System or Pancreas

Disorders of the Liver

Disorders of the Biliary Tract

MASTER HOME CARE PLANNING GUIDE
FOR CONDITIONS OF THE HEPATOBILIARY SYSTEM
AND PANCREAS

Pattern	Assessment Factors	Plan
1. Health management deficit	How long has the patient been acutely ill? Has the patient become weak and unable to care for self or others? Has the patient's employment been affected? Does the patient suffer from substance abuse such as alcohol?	Interview primary caregiver and patient. Involve social service.
2. Alteration in nutrition	Emphasis on nutritional status is indicated because of involvement of this system in nutrition.	See specific DRG.
3. Alteration in elimination	Digestive processes may be interrupted and there may be bowel elimination problems.	See specific DRG.
4. Activity and exercise	Assess level of home management deficit as *mild, moderate, severe, potential* or *chronic*.	
4a. Home maintenance management deficit		Interview patient and family to determine living arrangements, bathroom facilities, grocery supplies, transportation for follow-up, homemaker needs. Determine potential home management deficit taking into consideration: diagnosis and prognosis, level of care needed, ability and availability of caregiver.

5. Cognitive perceptual deficit		See specific DRG.
5a. Knowledge deficit related to self-care	Assess patient's ability to do self-care; assess level of understanding of signs and symptoms of complications. If patient's condition is related to alcohol abuse, assess patient's potential to be compliant in self-care.	
5b. Pain management	Assess patient's pain threshold and plan for pain control through comfort measures and diversional activities. Some pain medications cause spasm which will affect the biliary sphincters and some cannot be detoxified in a diseased liver. If the patient has alcoholic tendencies, potential for drug abuse or overuse must be assessed.	Review comfort measures for pain relief with patient and family. Discuss all real and potential problems of narcotic use in some patients. See specific DRG.
6. Alteration in self-perception and increased anxiety	Diseases of this system have relatively long LOS. Prognosis may be guarded or poor.	Allow patient and family to verbalize fears and refer to social service for counseling.
7. Coping tolerance	Length of time for recuperation will affect patient's responsibilities in caring for family or work related areas.	Communicate known facts to patient and family regarding estimated length of time patient will be incapacitated. See specific DRG.

DRG 191

MDC 07   **RW$ 4.1791**   **Surgical**   **Outlier Cutoff 41**   **Mean LOS 20.8**

Major Pancreas, Liver and Shunt Procedures

OPERATIVE PROCEDURES WITH POTENTIAL HOME CARE NEEDS

Hepatic lobectomy
Partial and total pancreatectomy

DETAILS TO CONSIDER

Long-term needs depend on amount of the organ removed, especially the pancreas. Patients undergoing surgery for liver or pancreas disease may have chronic disease states caused by complications.

POTENTIAL HOME CARE PROBLEMS	PLAN
1. Health management deficit potential related to need for long-term medical follow-up.	Assess patient's understanding of need for follow-up medical treatment and replacement medication.
2. Alteration in nutrition and metabolism secondary to pancreatic disease with potential for malabsorption of protein, carbohydrates and vitamin B_{12}.	Instruct patient about dietary restrictions, especially if patient is diabetic or has fat intolerance. Obtain specific diet order and provide instruction for patient and significant others.
3. Elimination problems.	Liver and pancreas play a role in digestion and elimination. Instruct the patient to seek medical attention if there is a change in color, consistency or frequency of bowel movements.
4. Pain control.	Assess patient's tolerance to pain. Instruct patient to seek medical attention for episodes of pain and to try to describe the type, location and progression of the pain so that the clinical problems can be more easily evaluated. Instruct the patient to avoid self-medication for pain since pain is an important sign in early detection of complications.

REFERRAL INFORMATION

Background information — communicate pertinent health history and prognosis, pertinent family situation and living arrangements. Current hospitalization history including complications — course of illness, including condition of wound and patient's level of ability regarding activities of daily living. Durable medical equipment — none needed unless assistive device needed for ambulation or bathing.

MDC 07   RW\$ 3.9197   Surgical   Outlier Cutoff 40   Mean LOS 20.1

Minor Pancreas, Liver and Shunt Procedures

OPERATIVE PROCEDURES WITH POTENTIAL HOME CARE NEEDS

Pancreatotomy
Pancreatic cyst marsupialization
Catheter drain pancreatic cyst
Choledochohepatic intubation

DETAILS TO CONSIDER

See **DRG 191.**

MDC 07   RW\$ 2.4513   Surgical   Outlier Cutoff 37   Mean LOS 17.3

Biliary Tract Procedure
Except Total Cholecystectomy – Age > = 70 and/or CC

OPERATIVE PROCEDURES WITH POTENTIAL HOME CARE NEEDS

Partial cholecystectomy
Common duct excision
Choledochoplasty
Percutaneous excision of common duct calculus

DETAILS TO CONSIDER

Patient is older than 70 or less than 70 with comorbidity or complications. Biliary tract disease can be caused by calculi or narrowing. These can be chronic or reoccurring problems.

POTENTIAL HOME CARE PROBLEMS	PLAN
1. Health management deficit secondary to age of patient or other illness.	Assess patient's ability to comply with health regime for other illness and assess impact of present surgery on patient's ability to care for self.
2. Alteration in nutrition.	Determine dietary change needed and instruct patient. Restriction in fat may be necessary. Stress importance of avoiding alcoholic beverages because of the effect on the biliary tract.
3. Pain control.	Spasm of bile ducts may cause pain. Instruct patient to seek medical attention for pain before taking nonprescription drugs.

REFERRAL INFORMATION

If patient was receiving home care services, reinstate service.

See **DRG 191.**

DRG 194

MDC 07	RW$ 1.9881	Surgical	Outlier Cutoff 34	Mean LOS 13.9

Biliary Tract Procedure
Except Total Cholecystectomy – Age < 70 w/o CC

See **DRG 193.**

DRG 195

MDC 07	RW$ 2.1690	Surgical	Outlier Cutoff 36	Mean LOS 16.0

Total Cholecystectomy with
Common Duct Exploration – Age > = 70 and/or CC

OPERATIVE PROCEDURES WITH POTENTIAL HOME CARE NEEDS

Same as **DRG 193.**

DETAILS TO CONSIDER

Age of patient is over 70 or under 70 but with comorbidity and/or complications. Comorbidity diagnoses which may increase long-term needs are: Diabetes (**DRG 294** and **295**); Circulatory System (**DRG 128, 134, 139**).

POTENTIAL HOME CARE PROBLEMS

PLAN

1. Alteration in nutrition.

Determine diet orders, especially for fat intolerance. Not all patients will be on a low fat diet. Do diet teaching for a well-balanced diet including the need for vitamins, especially the fat soluble ones (A, D and E). Inclusion of calcium especially for the female patient who is susceptible to osteoporosis.

2. Self-care deficit related to wound closure.

Assess condition of wound on discharge. If wound not completely closed, assess patient's and caregiver's ability to manage dressings.

3. Pain management.

The patient will have incisional pain and may need medication. Since large muscles are cut, patient will need to gradually increase activity. Common duct exploration may produce some spasm of the bile ducts resulting in pain. Instruct patient to call physician if any pain that is not incisional persists.

REFERRAL INFORMATION

None unless wound dressings or treatments cannot be done by patient or caregiver.

| MDC 07 | RW$ 2.0594 | Surgical | Outlier Cutoff 36 | Mean LOS 15.8 |

Total Cholecystectomy with
Common Duct Exploration – Age < 70 w/o CC

See **DRG 195.**

| MDC 07 | RW$ 1.4868 | Surgical | Outlier Cutoff 29 | Mean LOS 11.5 |

Total Cholecystectomy without
Common Duct Exploration – Age > = 70 and/or CC

See **DRG 195.**

| MDC 07 | RW$ 1.2752 | Surgical | Outlier Cutoff 24 | Mean LOS 10.1 |

Total Cholecystectomy without
Common Duct Exploration – Age < 70 w/o CC

See **DRG 195.**

DRG 199

MDC 07	RW$ 2.4574	Surgical	Outlier Cutoff 38	Mean LOS 17.9

Hepatobiliary Diagnostic Procedure for Malignancy

OPERATIVE PROCEDURES WITH POTENTIAL HOME CARE NEEDS

Transabdominal gastroscopy
Pancreatic biopsy
Laparotomy
Laparoscopy for diagnostic purposes

DETAILS TO CONSIDER

Follow-up needs depend directly on findings of the diagnostic test.

POTENTIAL HOME CARE PROBLEM

Lack of knowledge related to disease process.

PLAN

Determine patient's level of understanding of diagnosis if it is available.

REFERRAL INFORMATION

The need for referral is directly dependent on the prognosis. If there is a malignancy, the patient may need a referral immediately or after method of treatment of the malignancy has been planned or carried out. If the diagnosis is a malignant condition, make a referral to the home care nurse for home evaluation.

DRG 200

MDC 07	RW$ 2.5818	Surgical	Outlier Cutoff 35	Mean LOS 15.1

Hepatobiliary Diagnostic Procedure for Nonmalignancy

See **DRG 199**.

Other Hepatobiliary or Pancreas Operative Procedures

OPERATIVE PROCEDURES WITH POTENTIAL HOME CARE NEEDS

Percutaneous chordotomy
Duodenal incision
Adhesiolysis

DETAILS TO CONSIDER

Follow-up care will be similar to diagnosis in **DRGs 191, 193** and **195.**

Cirrhosis and Alcoholic Hepatitis

PRINCIPAL DIAGNOSIS WITH POTENTIAL HOME CARE NEEDS

Cirrhosis and alcoholic hepatitis

DETAILS TO CONSIDER

Cirrhosis and alcoholic hepatitis are chronic diffuse liver diseases which result in widespread disruption of liver function. The hospitalized patient with these chronic conditions will be very ill and may continue to be relatively ill at the time of discharge. *Not all* cirrhosis is caused by alcoholism.

POTENTIAL HOME CARE PROBLEMS

PLAN

1. Health management deficit.

Assess patient's ability to care for self and caregiver's ability to care for patient. Patient and caregiver should be instructed in need for compliance with all points of care including diet restrictions, medications and abstinence from alcohol, even if condition is not directly related to alcohol. Patient may fatigue very easily and also have neurological changes.

2. Alteration in nutrition and metabolism pattern.

A specific diet order will be needed. Factors such as anorexia, nausea, weight loss, vomiting, anemia, vitamin deficiencies, fluid retention, electrolyte imbalance must be considered when planning the patient's diet. Also, neurological involvement and the potential for hepatic coma secondary to protein metabolism must be considered.

3. Alteration in elimination.	Because of liver involvement and changes in nutrition, bowel elimination must be monitored. Urine amount and color should be monitored also. Patient and family should be instructed to watch for changes in stool and urine.
4. Deficit in activity tolerance.	Because of fatigue patient may be unable to carry out daily activities. Patient should be instructed in energy preserving methods.
5. Pain control.	Since many medications are detoxified in the liver the patient and caregiver must be instructed to be alert to using any medication.
6. Potential for skin breakdown.	Symptomatic relief of itching and instructions in skin care such as bathing and use of lotions should be reviewed with caregiver. Frequent changes in position are necessary; if the patient has ascities, he/she may need a hospital bed at home.

REFERRAL INFORMATION

If the patient cannot carry out activities of daily living, arrangements for home care nurse and a home health aide for personal care should be made. If the patient lives alone, arrangements for an extended care facility may be necessary for a period of time. A hospital bed, electric if patient can use controls, is indicated. A bedside commode and an ambulatory assistive device such as a walker may be needed.

DRG 203

MDC 07	RW$ 1.0937	Medical	Outlier Cutoff 28	Mean LOS 8.0

Malignancy of Hepatobiliary System or Pancreas

PRINCIPAL DIAGNOSIS WITH POTENTIAL HOME CARE NEEDS

Malignancy of the liver, bile ducts or pancreas

DETAILS TO CONSIDER

Patient will most likely be receiving either chemotherapy or some form of radiation as a method of treatment. The patient may have been treated surgically on another admission. The home care needs will vary depending on the prognosis, the stage of illness and the speed of disease progression. The patient may be terminal and the goal of care may be to give terminal care at home.

The level of care and details may be similar to **DRG 202.**

REFERRAL INFORMATION

If the goal of treatment is terminal care at home, make a referral for hospice care.

Disorders of Pancreas Except Malignancy

PRINCIPAL DIAGNOSES WITH POTENTIAL HOME CARE NEEDS

Mump pancreatitis
Pancreatic cyst
Pancreas anomalies
Injury to pancreas (closed and open)

DETAILS TO CONSIDER

Follow-up care of patients with disorders of the pancreas is very important. Acute pancreatitis can be a cause of death. Chronic pancreatitis, if not treated, can lead to debilitation.

Refer to **DRG 191.**

POTENTIAL HOME CARE PROBLEMS

PLAN

1. Self-care deficit.

Arrange assistance if patient cannot carry out activities of daily living.

2. Alteration in nutrition.

Nutritional needs are important in healing of acute pancreatitis. Patient must be encouraged to avoid alcoholic beverages.

REFERRAL INFORMATION

If patient or caregiver cannot carry out bathing or other activities of daily living, a referral for home care nurse and home health aide should be made. Meals-on-wheels may be indicated.

DRG 205

MDC 07	RW$ 1.0822	Medical	Outlier Cutoff 28	Mean LOS 7.9

Disorders of the Liver Except Malignancy, Cirrhosis or Alcoholic Hepatitis – Age > = 70 and/or CC

PRINCIPAL DIAGNOSES WITH POTENTIAL HOME CARE NEEDS

Viral hepatitis
Syphilitic liver
Hepatomegaly
Hepatic coma

DETAILS TO CONSIDER

Some of these diagnoses have long-term implications and require follow-up care and reporting to public health agencies. These diseases tend to progress in stages. An example is viral hepatitis which progresses from prodromal stage (3–4 days), icteric stage (6–8 weeks), and recovery stage (3–4 months). Syphilitic liver is usually a condition of tertiary syphilis. Hepatic coma is a late stage of liver disease. The home care needs will be directly related to the stage of illness.

Refer to **DRGs 191, 193, 199** and **202.**

DRG 206

MDC 07	RW$ 0.9247	Medical	Outlier Cutoff 27	Mean LOS 6.8

Disorders of the Liver Except Malignancy, Cirrhosis or Alcoholic Hepatitis – Age < 70 w/o CC

See **DRG 205.**

| MDC 07 | RW$ 0.8492 | Medical | Outlier Cutoff 27 | Mean LOS 6.6 |

Disorders of the Biliary Tract – Age > = 70 and/or CC

PRINCIPAL DIAGNOSES WITH POTENTIAL HOME CARE NEEDS

Fistula
Perforated gall bladder

DETAILS TO CONSIDER

A fistula from the biliary tract will allow the passage of bile or pancreatic digestive juices into other organs or spaces. This causes inflammation, tissue destruction and can lead to necrosis. The long-term needs of the patient will depend on the anatomical location of the fistula and the organs involved. A perforated gall bladder will allow the leakage of bile into the abdominal cavity, and if ruptured because of infection, it can also contaminate many organs.

Refer to **DRGs 196** and **198**.

REFERRAL INFORMATION

If the patient will be unable to carry out activities of daily living, refer for home care nurse and home health aide.

| MDC 07 | RW$ 0.7315 | Medical | Outlier Cutoff 24 | Mean LOS 5.5 |

Disorders of the Biliary Tract – Age < 70 w/o CC

See **DRG 207**.

8 MDC 08
DISEASES AND DISORDERS OF THE MUSCULOSKELETAL SYSTEM AND CONNECTIVE TISSUE

SURGICAL GROUPINGS (26 DRGs)

Major Joint Procedures
Hip and Femur Procedures
Amputations
Back and Neck Procedures
Biopsies
Wound Debridement and Skin Graft
Lower Extremities and Humerus Procedures
Knee Procedures
Upper Extremity Procedures
Foot Procedures
Soft Tissue Procedures
Ganglion Procedures
Hand Procedures
Local Excision/Removal of Internal Fixed Devices
Arthroscopy

MEDICAL GROUPINGS (22 DRGs)

Fractures of Femur, Hip and Pelvis
Sprains, Strains and Dislocations
Osteomyelitis
Pathological Fractures and Malignancy
Connective Tissue Disorders
Septic Arthritis
Medical Back Problems
Bone Diseases and Septic Arthropathy
Nonspecific Arthropathies
Signs and Symptoms
Tendonitis, Myositis and Bursitis
Aftercare
Fractures, Sprains, Strains and Dislocations

MASTER HOME CARE PLANNING GUIDE FOR CONDITIONS OF THE MUSCULOSKELETAL SYSTEM AND CONNECTIVE TISSUE

Pattern	Assessment Factors	Plan
1. Health management deficit	Assess age of patient and caregiver.	Interview caregiver and schedule visit to coincide with treatment caregiver will be required to do.
2. Alteration in nutrition	Assess patient's ability to prepare food and feed self if upper extremities are affected.	Refer to occupational therapy for help in meal preparation and methods for feeding self.
3. Alteration in elimination	Assess patient's ability to manage toileting because of transfer or ambulation problems. Determine location of bathroom facilities.	Refer to physical therapy for transfer and ambulation instruction. See specific DRG.
4. Activity and exercise deficit	Assess the effect of the patient's condition on ability to ambulate or carry out activities of daily living safely. The joint or limb involved will have a direct effect on the patient's home care needs.	See specific DRG.
5. Knowledge deficit related to self-care	Assess patient's ability to manage home environment with ambulation problems or impairment in carrying out activities of daily living.	Plan team conference with various therapies to determine patient's level of understanding.
6. Alteration in sleep-rest pattern	Assess home environment for location of bedroom.	If patient cannot safely climb stairs to bedroom, encourage relocation of bed to same level as kitchen.
7. Coping/stress compromise	Assess effect of onset of illness, especially if as a result of trauma.	Allow patient to verbalize fear.
8. Role-relationship disturbance	Assess effect of illness on ability to work or carry out family responsibilities.	Refer to social service for counseling if job or family responsibilities will not be met. Include family in conference to determine impact of illness on the total family.

Major Joint Procedures

OPERATIVE PROCEDURES WITH POTENTIAL HOME CARE NEEDS

Total replacement of the knee, hip
Replace femoral head
Limb reattachment

DETAILS TO CONSIDER

Joint replacements are frequently done because of arthritis and pain. They are usually scheduled procedures and patients have been able to plan for posthospital care. Limb reattachments are complicated by the traumatic nature of the condition.

POTENTIAL HOME CARE PROBLEMS

1. Activity exercise deficit.

2. Knowledge deficit related to incision/wound care.

PLAN

Evaluate patient's ability to ambulate, interview for home arrangements for sleep, meals and toileting. Evaluate patient's ability to carry out activities of daily living if upper extremity is involved.

Instruct patient in incision care and signs/symptoms of infection. If patient has open wound instruct in care and refer to home care nurse.

REFERRAL INFORMATION

Patient may need physical therapy in the home to teach ambulation, joint mobility and safety. Patient should have raised toilet seat or adjustable commode for hip surgery. Safety rails and removal of area rugs at home should be discussed.

Patient may also need seat-lift chair for assistance in getting out of a chair, or stairway elevator if home environment cannot be adapted and climbing stairs unsafe. These are expensive items so the need should be validated carefully.

Limb reattachment surgery usually requires long-term care and follow-up. Patient may be unable to return to usual activities for a long period of time. A referral to social services is indicated.

DRG 210

MDC 08	RW$ 2.0833	Surgical	Outlier Cutoff 38	Mean LOS 17.8

Hip and Femur Procedures
Except Major Joint – Age $\geq$ 70 and/or CC

OPERATIVE PROCEDURES WITH POTENTIAL HOME CARE NEEDS

Open reduction of fractured head of femur with use of various hardware

DETAILS TO CONSIDER

The patient is over 70 or has a complication or comorbidity.

POTENTIAL HOME CARE PROBLEMS	PLAN
1a. Alteration in activity ambulation.	Assess patient's weight-bearing status and need for assistive device such as cane or walker. Check with physician to determine estimated length of time for guarded ambulation. This will be, in part, determined by the type of device used. Assess patient's ability to flex hip to determine need for raised toilet seat.
1b. Decrease in muscle strength secondary to bedrest.	Assess patient's need for strengthening exercises and confer with physical therapist.

REFERRAL INFORMATION

Continued physical therapy after discharge for ambulation and muscle strengthening should be arranged. Also, an evaluation of safety in the home is needed if patient lives in a home where there are steps. If there is an open wound, incomplete healing of the incision, or the comorbidity illness needs attention because patient has been hospitalized, then refer to a home care nurse.

DRG 211

MDC 08	RW$ 1.9530	Surgical	Outlier Cutoff 36	Mean LOS 15.9

Hip and Femur Procedures
Except Major Joint – Age 18–69 w/o CC

OPERATIVE PROCEDURE WITH POTENTIAL HOME CARE NEEDS

Open reduction of fracture of head of femur using various hardware

DETAILS TO CONSIDER

Refer to **DRG 210**.

MDC 08   RW$ 1.7132   Surgical   Outlier Cutoff 31   Mean LOS 11.1

Hip and Femur Procedures Except Major Joint – Age 0–17

OPERATIVE PROCEDURES WITH POTENTIAL HOME CARE NEEDS

Open reduction of fracture of head of femur with various hardware
Length change procedure

DETAILS TO CONSIDER

See **DRG 210.** The reader is referred to pediatric texts for more information.

DRG 213

MDC 08   RW$ 2.1315   Surgical   Outlier Cutoff 34   Mean LOS 14.3

Amputations for Musculoskeletal System and Connective Tissue Disorders

OPERATIVE PROCEDURES WITH POTENTIAL HOME CARE NEEDS

Amputations of the hand and arm
Amputations of the foot
Amputations of the leg: above the knee amputation; below the knee amputation

DETAILS TO CONSIDER

The age of the patient will have a direct effect on the need for referral. The reason for the amputation, such as trauma or peripheral vascular disease, will also have a direct effect on the patient's home care needs.

For hand injuries see **DRG 441.**

POTENTIAL HOME CARE PROBLEMS

PLAN

1. Self-care deficit secondary to amputation.

Evaluate patient's ability to ambulate and carry out activities of daily living. Utilize occupational physical therapist for activity plan.

2. Lack of knowledge related to care of stump and/or prosthesis.

With the patient and caregiver, teach care of stump and inform patient of plans for the prosthesis since the patient may be discharged prior to fitting of permanent prosthesis.

3. Potential coping deficit.

Assess patient's level of acceptance of condition.

REFERRAL INFORMATION

A referral to a home care agency should be made. Referral should include pertinent history about the reason for the procedure; patient's and caregiver's level of understanding of care and plans for care; patient's and family's level of acceptance of condition.

DRG 214

MDC 08	RW$ 1.8427	Surgical	Outlier Cutoff 36	Mean LOS 15.6

Back and Neck Procedures – Age > = 70 and/or CC

OPERATIVE PROCEDURES WITH POTENTIAL HOME CARE NEEDS

Fusion procedures
Vertebral fracture repair

DETAILS TO CONSIDER

The home care needs will depend on the extent of the injury to the spinal cord as a result of the vertebral fracture. If there is injury to the spinal cord and the patient becomes paraplegic or quadriplegic, a multidisciplinary team approach is needed. Patients with these injuries should be referred for rehabilitation follow-up. If there is no injury to the spinal cord, referrals are not usually necessary unless there is an unhealed wound.

DRG 215

MDC 08	RW$ 1.4920	Surgical	Outlier Cutoff 33	Mean LOS 13.0

Back and Neck Procedures – Age < 70 w/o CC

See DRG 214.

DRG 216

MDC 08	RW$ 1.5596	Surgical	Outlier Cutoff 31	Mean LOS 11.3

Biopsies of the Musculoskeletal System and Connective Tissue

OPERATIVE PROCEDURES WITH POTENTIAL HOME CARE NEEDS

Skull biopsy
Facial bone
Chest cage
Humerus or other bone biopsy

DETAILS TO CONSIDER

The patient's home care needs will depend on the outcome of the biopsy and the patient's general health status, especially if the patient is weak or is recovering from pathological fractures.

Wound Debridement and Skin Graft, Except Hand, for Musculoskeletal and Connective Tissue Disease

OPERATIVE PROCEDURES WITH POTENTIAL HOME CARE NEEDS

Free skin graft
Full-thickness graft
Pedicle graft

DETAILS TO CONSIDER

The patient's extended needs will depend on the areas of the body involved. If the legs are involved and the patient is immobilized, extensive home care will be needed.

POTENTIAL HOME CARE PROBLEM

Lack of knowledge related to care of graft and/or donor site.

PLAN

Teach patient and caregiver procedure. Determine supplies and equipment that will be needed for care.

REFERRAL INFORMATION

Refer for nursing care to instruct patient and caregiver in wound management at home, for monitoring healing and signs/symptoms of infection. If patient is immobilized and cannot do self-care or meal preparation, evaluate home health needs. Refer patient to medical supply company for purchasing of wound-care supplies.

DRG 218

MDC 08	RW$ 1.4250	Surgical	Outlier Cutoff 31	Mean LOS 10.9

Lower Extremity and Humerus Procedure Except Hip, Foot, Femur – Age > = 70 and/or CC

OPERATIVE PROCEDURES WITH POTENTIAL HOME CARE NEEDS

Osteotomy
Internal fixation device to humerus
Ankle fusion
Implant leg prosthesis
Open reduction tibia-fibula fracture

DETAILS TO CONSIDER

Patient is over 70 or has a complication or comorbidity. The home care needs will depend on the effect of the surgery on the patient's other diseases or on the complication.

POTENTIAL HOME CARE PROBLEMS	PLAN
1. Decreased activity secondary to:	Assess patient's ability to carry out activities of
1a. Immobilization of upper extremity.	daily living such as bathing, dressing, preparing and eating meals.
1b. Limited use of lower extremity.	Assess patient's ability to ambulate and need for assistive devices such as crutches or walker.

REFERRAL INFORMATION

Refer to home health agency if complication or comorbidity is significant enough to make patient unable to ambulate or carry out activities of daily living.

DRG 219

MDC 08	RW$ 1.0790	Surgical	Outlier Cutoff 27	Mean LOS 8.3

Lower Extremity and Humerus Procedure Except Hip, Foot, Femur – Age 18–69 w/o CC

OPERATIVE PROCEDURES WITH POTENTIAL HOME CARE NEEDS

Osteotomy
Internal fixation device of humerus
Length change of humerus
Ankle fusion
Implant leg prosthesis
Open reduction of tibia-fibula fracture

DETAILS TO CONSIDER

The home care needs will depend on the patient's ability to carry out activities of daily living or ambulation.

See **DRG 218.**

| MDC 08 | RW\$ 0.9339 | Surgical | Outlier Cutoff 25 | Mean LOS 5.3 |

Lower Extremity and Humerus Procedures
Except Hip, Foot, Femur – Age 0–17

See **DRGs 212** and **219**. The reader is referred to pediatric texts for more information.

| MDC 08 | RW\$ 1.2727 | Surgical | Outlier Cutoff 28 | Mean LOS 8.3 |

Knee Procedures – Age $\geq$ 70 and/or CC

OPERATIVE PROCEDURES WITH POTENTIAL HOME CARE NEEDS

Patellar procedures, including patellectomy
Arthrodesis of knee
Knee synovectomy

DETAILS TO CONSIDER

Patient is over 70 and has comorbidity and/or a complication.

POTENTIAL HOME CARE PROBLEM

Decrease in activity secondary to knee procedure.

PLAN

Assess patient's ability to ambulate safely. Assess need for assistive device such as crutches, cane or walker.

REFERRAL INFORMATION

Refer for follow-up physical therapy for joint mobility and ambulation if ordered by the physician. If patient's comorbidity has compromised his/her ability to carry out activities of daily living, refer for nursing evaluation.

| MDC 08 | RW\$ 0.9897 | Surgical | Outlier Cutoff 26 | Mean LOS 6.4 |

Knee Procedures – Age $<$ 70 w/o CC

See **DRG 221**.

DRG 223

| MDC 08 | RW$ 1.0723 | Surgical | Outlier Cutoff 27 | Mean LOS 6.9 |

Upper Extremity Procedures
Except Humerus and Hand – Age > = 70 and/or CC

OPERATIVE PROCEDURES WITH POTENTIAL HOME CARE NEEDS

Procedures on radius and ulna
Dislocation of shoulder
Elbow or shoulder synovectomy
Arthodesis of shoulder
Rotator cuff repair

DETAILS TO CONSIDER

Patient is over 70 and has comorbidity and/or a complication. Long-term needs will depend on the effect of these on the patient's ability to carry out activities of daily living.

POTENTIAL HOME CARE PROBLEM

Alteration in activity secondary to upper extremity limitation.

PLAN

Assess patient's ability to bathe, dress and feed self. Assess patient's balance and safety in ambulation.

REFERRAL INFORMATION

If patient's general condition is affected by procedure, refer for home evaluation.

DRG 224

| MDC 08 | RW$ 0.8952 | Surgical | Outlier Cutoff 24 | Mean LOS 5.6 |

Upper Extremity Procedures
Except Humerus and Hand – Age < 70 w/o CC

See **DRG 223**.

MDC 08   **RW$ 0.6476**   **Surgical**   **Outlier Cutoff 15**   **Mean LOS 4.8**

Foot Procedures

OPERATIVE PROCEDURES WITH POTENTIAL HOME CARE NEEDS

Bunionectomy
Tarsal length change
Repair of fractures
Debridement of open fracture of metatarsus or toe
Achillotenotomy
Toe amputation
Toe reattachment
Fusion of toe

DETAILS TO CONSIDER

Patient's long-term needs will depend on weight bearing status.

POTENTIAL HOME CARE PROBLEM

Alteration in activity secondary to foot procedure.

PLAN

Assess effect on ambulation and need for crutch, cane or walker.

REFERRAL INFORMATION

If patient's ability to carry out activities of daily living is compromised, refer for home assessment and evaluation of need for assistance.

MDC 08   **RW$ 0.7984**   **Surgical**   **Outlier Cutoff 25**   **Mean LOS 5.1**

Soft Tissue Procedures – Age > = 70 and/or CC

OPERATIVE PROCEDURES WITH POTENTIAL HOME CARE NEEDS

Synovectomy
Myotomy
Bursotomy/bursectomy
Muscle transfer/transplant
Insertion of skeletal muscle stimulator
Tendon or muscle reattachment

DETAILS TO CONSIDER

Patient is over 70 and has a complication or comorbidity. Home care needs will be directly related to muscle or soft tissues involved as well as on the effect on the patient's ability to ambulate or carry out activities of daily living.

REFERRAL INFORMATION

See DRG 218.

DRG 227

| MDC 08 | RW$ 0.6337 | Surgical | Outlier Cutoff 18 | Mean LOS 4.2 |

Soft Tissue Procedures – Age < 70 w/o CC

See **DRG 226.**

DRG 228

| MDC 08 | RW$ 0.3626 | Surgical | Outlier Cutoff 7 | Mean LOS 2.2 |

Ganglion (Hand) Procedures

OPERATIVE PROCEDURES WITH POTENTIAL HOME CARE NEEDS

Procedures on the hand

DETAILS TO CONSIDER

Ganglion procedures are usually done on an elective basis allowing patient an opportunity to plan for follow-up care. Usual course is for some limitation of wrist use for approximately 3 weeks.

DRG 229

| MDC 08 | RW$ 0.5998 | Surgical | Outlier Cutoff 14 | Mean LOS 3.4 |

Hand Procedures Except Ganglion

OPERATIVE PROCEDURES WITH POTENTIAL HOME CARE NEEDS

Carpal tunnel release
Bone graft
Closed or open reduction of fracture
Wrist synovectomy
Hand skin graft
Syndactyly correction
Thumb reconstruction

DETAILS TO CONSIDER

Some hand procedures in this DRG are done on elective admissions.

See **DRG 228.**

POTENTIAL HOME CARE PROBLEM

Alteration in activity secondary to inability to use hand.

PLAN

Assess patient's ability to do activities of daily living. Confer with occupational therapist for assistive devices.

REFERRAL INFORMATION

If patient is unable to carry out activities of daily living, refer to home health agency for occupational therapy and assistive devices for the home.

DRG 230

MDC 08	RW$ 1.3594	Surgical	Outlier Cutoff 29	Mean LOS 8.9

Local Excision and Removal of Internal Fixation Devices of the Hip and Femur

OPERATIVE PROCEDURES WITH POTENTIAL HOME CARE NEEDS

Local excision and removal of internal fixation devices of the hip and femur

DETAILS TO CONSIDER

See **DRGs 209** and **210**. Length of time from insertion to removal of fixation device varies.

POTENTIAL HOME CARE PROBLEM

Alteration in ambulation.

PLAN

Assess patient's ability to ambulate safely.

REFERRAL INFORMATION

If the patient has less mobility at time of discharge than on admission, refer for physical therapy.

DRG 231

MDC 08   **RW$ 0.9519**   **Surgical**   **Outlier Cutoff 25**   **Mean LOS 5.3**

Local Excision and Removal of Internal Fixation Devices Except Hip and Femur

OPERATIVE PROCEDURES WITH POTENTIAL HOME CARE NEEDS

Removal of fixation devices from: the skull, tibia/fibula, chest cage, humerus, radius and ulna

DETAILS TO CONSIDER

Length of time from insertion to removal of fixture varies.

POTENTIAL HOME CARE PROBLEMS	PLAN
Alteration in activity: ambulation and ADLs	Assess patient's ability to ambulate safely and ability to carry out activities of daily living.

REFERRAL INFORMATION

If patient is less mobile at time of discharge than on admission, refer for physical therapy for ambulation training or to occupational therapy for training in activities of daily living.

DRG 232

MDC 08   **RW$ 0.6063**   **Surgical**   **Outlier Cutoff 15**   **Mean LOS 3.6**

Arthroscopy

OPERATIVE PROCEDURES WITH POTENTIAL HOME CARE NEEDS

Arthroscopy — examination of the interior of a joint with an arthroscope.

DETAILS TO CONSIDER

This procedure is frequently done on an outpatient basis.

MDC 08   **RW$ 1.7737**   **Surgical**   **Outlier Cutoff 33**   **Mean LOS 13.1**

Other Musculoskeletal System and Connective Tissue Operating Room Procedures – Age > = 70 and/or CC

OPERATIVE PROCEDURES WITH POTENTIAL HOME CARE NEEDS

Craniectomy
Rhinoplasty
Facial bone repair
Pectus deformity repair
Mandible surgery

DETAILS TO CONSIDER

Procedures in this DRG vary greatly; therefore the home care needs will vary also. The patient will be over 70 and have a comorbidity or complication. The needs will depend on the effect of the surgery on the comorbidity and the complication.

POTENTIAL HOME CARE PROBLEMS

1. Alteration in activity and ability to carry out activities of daily living.

2. Potential alteration in nutrition secondary to surgery of facial bones.

PLAN

Assess patient's ability to carry out activities of daily living.

Assess patient's ability to chew and swallow.

REFERRAL INFORMATION

If patient's status regarding activities of daily living indicates, a referral for occupational therapy may be necessary. If the patient is unable to chew food, referral for liquid nutritional supplement is indicated. A consultation with a nutritionist is also indicated if the patient is on a special diet.

MDC 08   **RW$ 1.2454**   **Surgical**   **Outlier Cutoff 28**   **Mean LOS 8.2**

Other Musculoskeletal System and Connective Tissue Operating Room Procedures – Age < 70 w/o CC

See **DRG 233.**

DRG 235

MDC 08　　　**RW$ 1.7586**　　　**Medical**　　　**Outlier Cutoff 34**　　　**Mean LOS 13.6**

Fractures of the Femur

DIAGNOSES WITH POTENTIAL HOME CARE NEEDS

Closed fracture of the shaft, condyle or lower femur epiphysis

DETAILS TO CONSIDER

Patient may be discharged in a hip spica cast or a cast brace. Plans will depend upon whether patient will be ambulatory with an assistive device such as a walking spica or cast brace, or if they are discharged in full spica and are nonambulatory. The age of the patient will also have direct effect on home care needs.

POTENTIAL HOME CARE PROBLEMS
(*If Ambulatory*)

PLAN

1. Alteration in activity — mobility.

The patient will be ambulatory with assistive device (walker or crutches). Weight-bearing status will be according to doctor's orders. Assess patient's independence at home in activities of daily living and need for equipment, such as being elevated over the toilet, and safety bars.

2. Knowledge deficit related to management in a cast.

Instruct patient in cast care, such as keeping cast dry and knowing how to recognize signs of circulatory impairment.

POTENTIAL HOME CARE PROBLEMS
(*If Nonambulatory*)

PLAN

1. Alteration in mobility.

Patient should exercise unaffected extremities to maintain circulation and strengthen muscles and assist in self-care as much as allowed by cast. Patient should use side rails and trapeze to change positions.

2. Potential for skin breakdown.

Instruct patient and family in the plan of care including need for patient to be turned prone at least twice a day and to sleep prone as much as possible at night. Inspect skin for signs of skin breakdown. Instruct caregiver in use of bed pan, especially the need to protect both cast and patient's skin.

3. Alteration in elimination.

Review with patient and caregiver the need for a well-balanced diet with high fiber content and adequate fluids to avoid constipation. The physician should be contacted if a laxative is needed.

4. Alteration in nutrition

Because of the pressure of the cast the patient may be more comfortable with small, frequent meals.

5. Safety hazard.

Because the patient is immobile the Fire Department should be notified in writing regarding the patient's status and the exact location of the patient in the house so the patient can be reached immediately in case of an emergency. PATIENT SHOULD NEVER BE LEFT ALONE IN THE HOME!

DETAILS TO CONSIDER

If patient is to be discharged nonambulatory in a spica cast, the equipment needed is a hospital bed, side rails and trapeze. Home care nursing referral should be made for supervision and assessment of family member or other responsible person's ability to care for the patient with a hip spica cast. Home assessment should be made prior to discharge to facilitate care in the home.

DRG 236

MDC 08	RW$ 1.3855	Medical	Outlier Cutoff 32	Mean LOS 11.9

Fractures of Hip and Pelvis

DIAGNOSES WITH POTENTIAL HOME CARE NEEDS

Fracture of pelvis, such as acetabulum and pelvis
Femoral neck fractures such as subtrochanteric or intratrochanteric fractures

DETAILS TO CONSIDER

Patients with pelvic fractures may be ambulatory with crutches, walker or a cane. Fractures of the hip treated without surgery will require bedrest or activity restrictions such as bed-to-chair movement for an extended period of time.

DRG 237

MDC 08	RW$ 0.7929	Medical	Outlier Cutoff 26	Mean LOS 6.4

Sprains, Strains and Dislocations of Hip, Pelvis and Thigh

DIAGNOSES WITH POTENTIAL HOME CARE NEEDS

Sprains, strains and dislocations of hip, pelvis and thigh

DETAILS TO CONSIDER

Patients will be ambulatory with crutches or walker. Length of time will depend on doctor's instructions. Age factor will greatly influence home care needs. A sprain is an incomplete tearing of the capsule or ligaments of a joint. A strain is a traumatic injury in which the ligament or tenden is used beyond its usual limits.

REFERRAL INFORMATION

If patient is being discharged ambulating with a walker or crutch, refer as your would a post-op hip surgery patient.

See **DRGs 210** and **211.**

DRG 238

MDC 08   **RW$ 1.5511**   **Medical**   **Outlier Cutoff 32**   **Mean LOS 12.3**

Osteomyelitis

DIAGNOSES WITH POTENTIAL HOME CARE NEEDS

Osteomyelitis of limb bones

DETAILS TO CONSIDER

This condition may be acute or chronic. Chronic osteomyelitis is subject to sporadic flare-ups of acute symptoms. Acute episodes require in-hospital treatment. Patient may be discharged on IV antibiotic therapy. Plans can be made for either outpatient or home IV antibiotic therapy.

In outpatient IV antibiotic therapy, the plan includes home administration of the medication and outpatient visits to a clinic or hospital for change of the IV site and additional instruction. In home IV antibiotic therapy, the medication is delivered and the IV site and additional education is done in the home.

Some programs utilize a combination of the two. For example, the patient may return to the clinic for the site change and education and have the medications and equipment delivered by a company that specializes in home IV antibiotic therapy. The choice of therapy depends on several factors, such as availability of an outpatient program, patient's vein status and patient's home-bound status.

POTENTIAL HOME CARE PROBLEMS

PLAN

1. Lack of knowledge related to IV therapy.

Assess caregiver's and patient's ability to learn and carry out the therapy. Patients who live alone should not be sent home on IV therapy without a thorough evaluation of their ability to do the procedure and to receive help from a close neighbor.

2. Access to vein site.

Prior to instituting the plan, an assessment of the vein status should be done. If continuous access is questionable, the physician may elect to insert a central vein line. Several styles are available.

3. Financial considerations.

Third party reimbursement, including Medicare, for this type of therapy must be investigated. Coverage varies from policy to policy. Since this is relatively expensive, the patient must be informed of extent of coverage and patient's financial responsibility.

REFERRAL INFORMATION

The person making the referral should consider the vein status, type and duration of therapy, living situation and home-bound status of the patient and develop an individualized plan for the patient. The insurance and/or Medicare coverage should be evaluated carefully, and the best possible plan or combination of plans made.

MDC 08   **RW$ 1.0979**   **Medical**   **Outlier Cutoff 29**   **Mean LOS 9.2**

Pathological Fractures and Musculoskeletal and Connective Tissue Malignancy

DIAGNOSIS WITH POTENTIAL HOME CARE NEEDS

Pathological fractures and musculoskeletal and connective tissue malignancy

DETAILS TO CONSIDER

Home care management and needs will vary greatly according to the area affected, age of the patient and stage of the malignancy. The fracture may be treated by casting or bracing. In pathological vertebral fractures, the patient should be assessed for possible development of neurological deficits such as paraparesis or paraplegia.

MDC 08   **RW$ 0.9709**   **Medical**   **Outlier Cutoff 29**   **Mean LOS 8.6**

Connective Tissue Disorders – Age $>=$ 70 and/or CC

DIAGNOSES WITH POTENTIAL HOME CARE NEEDS

Reiter's disease
Amyloidosis
Raynaud's disease
Polyarteritis nodosa
Felty's syndrome
Polymyalgia rheumatica
Rheumatic arthritis

DETAILS TO CONSIDER

Home care needs will be determined by the organ or area involved, the severity of the disorder and the patient's ability to perform activities of daily living. Each patient will need individual assessment and planning.

DRG 241

MDC 08	RW$ 0.9048	Medical	Outlier Cutoff 28	Mean LOS 8.0

Connective Tissue Disorders – Age < 70 w/o CC

See **DRG 240**.

DRG 242

MDC 08	RW$ 1.5880	Medical	Outlier Cutoff 31	Mean LOS 11.2

Septic Arthritis

DIAGNOSES WITH POTENTIAL HOME CARE NEEDS

Viral arthritis
Bacterial arthritis
Helminth (worm) arthritis
Mycotic (fungal) arthritis
Pyogenic arthritis
Inflammatory arthritis

DETAILS TO CONSIDER

Home care needs will depend upon the severity, the joints involved and whether this is a long-standing problem and degenerative changes have occurred. Immobilization may be required. Patients can be expected to be on oral or IV antibiotic therapy. Physical therapy may be ordered after subsidence of acute episode if there are residual effects.

MDC 08 **RW$ 0.7551** **Medical** **Outlier Cutoff 28** **Mean LOS 7.5**

Medical Back Problems

DIAGNOSES WITH POTENTIAL HOME CARE NEEDS

Spondylolysis
Sacroiliitis
Disc displacement
Postlaminectomy syndrome
Curvature of the spine
Dislocated vertebrae
Fracture of vertebrae
Sprain of back

DETAILS TO CONSIDER

Home care needs depend upon the severity of the problem. Casting or bracing will be necessary for some disorders. Needs will also depend upon whether disability interferes with ability to perform activities of daily living. Physical therapy may be ordered for some conditions.

POTENTIAL HOME CARE PROBLEMS

PLAN

1. Health management deficit secondary to long-term needs.

Assess effect of long-term health problem on patient's ability to care for self or others.

2. Alteration in pain management.

Establish pain control plan with physician, patient and others as needed, such as pharmacist or physical therapist. Pain control in back problems will be a long-standing problem. The potential for drug tolerance and need for changes in dose and types of drugs should be discussed.

3. Alteration in activity-exercise.

If the patient's physician prescribes traction at home, instruct patient in all aspects of traction, including mechanism of the equipment, proper alignment and skin care.

4. Alteration in self-perception.

Assess impact of back problem on lifestyle and work situation. If patient will need to change lifestyle or be unable to assume usual role in the family, refer for counseling.

REFERRAL INFORMATION

Patients with medical back problems are usually not home-bound and can usually ambulate with minimal assistance. Those needing intermittent traction only can receive instructions prior to discharge and from the physician. Home care companies that supply home traction service can set up the device prescribed and give the patient and family instructions on safety. If the patient is incapacitated and cannot carry out activities of daily living, a referral for a home care nurse is indicated.

DRG 244

Bone Diseases and Septic Arthropathy – Age $>= 70$ and/or CC

DIAGNOSES WITH POTENTIAL HOME CARE NEEDS

Arthritis
Osteomalacia
Viral arthritis
Osteoarthrosis

DETAILS TO CONSIDER

The home care needs in the broad spectrum of this category will depend upon the age of the patient and the extent of disability involved. The choice of therapy will have an effect on the long-term needs.

POTENTIAL HOME CARE PROBLEMS

PLAN

1. Health management deficit secondary to limited mobility.

Assess effect of joint involvement on activities of daily living. Needs vary greatly depending on joints. Lower limb joints can affect ambulation and upper limb joints can affect ability to do manual activities.

2. Alteration in elimination pattern.

Assess patient's ability to ambulate to bathroom and carry out hygiene needs after toileting.

3. Alteration in activity/exercise pattern.

Assess patient's ability to ambulate and need for assistive devices, safety rails. Assess need for physical therapy for instruction in ambulation and stair-climbing, especially if patient has steps in the home.

4. Knowledge deficit related to disease process and potential side effects of therapy.

Instruct patient and family in disease process and signs/symptoms of untoward effects of drugs and the potential drug interaction with over-the-counter drugs.

REFERRAL INFORMATION

If the patient is limited in activities of daily living, refer to a home health agency for evaluation of home setting. If patient previously received home care services, notify the agency of any changes in patient's condition.

| MDC 08 | RW$ 0.7177 | Medical | Outlier Cutoff 26 | Mean LOS 6.3 |

Bone Disease and Septic Arthropathy – Age < 70 w/o CC

DIAGNOSES WITH POTENTIAL HOME CARE NEEDS

Juvenile osteochondrosis

See **DRG 244.**

DETAILS TO CONSIDER

Juvenile patients will be immobilized or in bed for long periods. Specific intervention is determined by physician's preference and stage of progression at the time of diagnosis. Needs will vary accordingly and may involve rest, traction, cast or brace application. The reader is referred to pediatric texts for additional information.

See **DRG 244.**

| MDC 08 | RW$ 0.7147 | Medical | Outlier Cutoff 27 | Mean LOS 6.8 |

Nonspecific Arthropathies

DIAGNOSES WITH POTENTIAL HOME CARE NEEDS

Polyarthritis
Monoarthritis

DETAILS TO CONSIDER

Needs will vary according to the number and severity of the joints involved, how the disease affects the patient's ability to perform activities of daily living and the patient's age. May need to have physical therapy in the home.

See **DRG 244.**

DRG 247

MDC 08	RW$ 0.6559	Medical	Outlier Cutoff 26	Mean LOS 5.8

Signs and Symptoms of Musculoskeletal System and Connective Tissue

DIAGNOSES WITH POTENTIAL HOME CARE NEEDS

Joint pain
Joint stiffness
Difficulty walking
Pain in limb
Somatic dysfunction

DETAILS TO CONSIDER

Needs will be determined by extent of pain and disability as well as the ability to perform activities of daily living. The length of stay for conditions in this DRG is relatively short. The referral needs for these patients will include arrangements for follow-up medical care.

See **DRG 244.**

DRG 248

MDC 08	RW$ 0.6136	Medical	Outlier Cutoff 24	Mean LOS 5.4

Tendonitis, Myositis and Bursitis

DIAGNOSES WITH POTENTIAL HOME CARE NEEDS

Tendonitis
Myositis
Bursitis

DETAILS TO CONSIDER

These are usually temporary, treatable conditions. Symptoms vary according to the location. In acute phase there may be temporary compromise in activities of daily living, but following treatment the patient should be at the same level of functioning as prior to admission.

MDC 08	RW$ 1.0203	Medical	Outlier Cutoff 28	Mean LOS 7.6

Aftercare, Musculoskeletal System and Connective Tissue

DIAGNOSES WITH POTENTIAL HOME CARE NEEDS

Fitting artificial limb
Complication of reattachment procedure

DETAILS TO CONSIDER

The home care needs will need to be planned individually, depending on the stage of therapy. The patient will need a referral for a long-term rehabilitation program and medical follow-up.

See **Master Care Plan.**

MDC 08	RW$ 0.7428	Medical	Outlier Cutoff 26	Mean LOS 6.0

Fractures, Sprains, Strains and Dislocations of Forearm, Hand, Foot – Age > = 70 and/or CC

DIAGNOSES WITH POTENTIAL HOME CARE NEEDS

Fractures, sprains, strains, and dislocations of forearm, hand, foot

DETAILS TO CONSIDER

Age of the patient and comorbidity may require casting, soft casting or Ace bandage.

POTENTIAL HOME CARE PROBLEMS / PLAN

POTENTIAL HOME CARE PROBLEMS	PLAN
1. Alteration in ambulation.	Assess patient's weight-bearing status and ability to ambulate safely with assistive device in the home, especially in cases of lower limb involvement.
2. Alteration in ability to perform activities of daily living.	Assess patient's ability to perform activities of daily living and provide the necessary equipment and help with those activities.

REFERRAL INFORMATION

These conditions result in temporary limitations and may not require assistance. However, the condition may interfere significantly in the ability to manage, especially in the frail elderly or those living alone. In these cases a referral for home care nursing is indicated.

DRG 251

MDC 08	RW$ 0.5964	Medical	Outlier Cutoff 24	Mean LOS 4.2

Fractures, Sprains, Strains and Dislocations of Forearm, Hand, Foot – Age 18–69 w/o CC

See **DRG 250**.

DRG 252

MDC 08	RW$ 0.3533	Medical	Outlier Cutoff 7	Mean LOS 1.8

Fractures, Sprains, Strains and Dislocations of Forearm, Hand, Foot – Age 0–17

See **DRG 250**.

The reader is also referred to pediatric texts for additional information.

DRG 253

MDC 08	RW$ 0.7466	Medical	Outlier Cutoff 27	Mean LOS 6.6

Fractures, Sprains, Strains and Dislocations of Upper Arm, Lower Leg, Except Foot – Age > = 70 and/or CC

DETAILS TO CONSIDER

Length of time of required immobilization will have a direct effect on home care needs.

See **DRG 250**.

MDC 08	RW$ 0.6258	Medical	Outlier Cutoff 25	Mean LOS 5.3

Fractures, Sprains, Strains and Dislocations of Upper Arm, Lower Leg, Except Foot – Age 18–69 w/o CC

See **DRG 250** and **DRG 253**.

MDC 08	RW$ 0.4687	Medical	Outlier Cutoff 15	Mean LOS 2.9

Fractures, Sprains, Strains and Dislocations of Upper Arm, Lower Leg, Except Foot – Age 0–17

See **DRG 250**.

The reader is referred to pediatric texts for additional information.

MDC 08	RW$ 0.8706	Medical	Outlier Cutoff 27	Mean LOS 6.5

Other Diagnoses of Musculoskeletal System and Connective Tissue

DIAGNOSES WITH POTENTIAL HOME CARE NEEDS

Recurrent dislocation
Hallux valgus deformity
Congenital bone defect
Osteogenesis imperfecta

DETAILS TO CONSIDER

Home care needs and nursing needs in this broad category will depend upon the diagnosis, severity of involvement and age. Many are chronic conditions needing regular medical care. Determine the effect of hospitalization on long-term needs. Variations in pre-hospital plans may be needed. Communicate changes to appropriate agency and/or caregiver.

9 MDC 09
DISEASES AND DISORDERS OF THE SKIN, SUBCUTANEOUS TISSUE AND BREAST

SURGICAL GROUPINGS (14 DRGs)

Mastectomy for Malignancy

Breast Procedure for Nonmalignancy

Breast Biopsy and Local Excision

Skin Grafts

Perianal and Pilonidal Procedures

Plastic Procedures

Other OR Procedures

MEDICAL GROUPINGS (14 DRGs)

Skin Ulcers

Major Skin Disorders

Malignant and Nonmalignant Breast Disorders

Cellulitis

Trauma

Minor Skin Disorders

MASTER HOME CARE PLANNING GUIDE
FOR DISEASES AND DISORDERS OF THE SKIN,
SUBCUTANEOUS TISSUE AND BREAST

Pattern	Assessment Factors	Plan
1. Health management deficit	The location of the wound, the complexity of the dressing, if any, and the availability of a caregiver who can do wound care should all be considered in making the home care plan.	If the patient or caregiver cannot do the wound care, refer for home nursing services. See specific DRG.
2. Alteration in nutrition	Assess patient's ability to buy groceries and prepare meals. Adequate nutrition is vital in the healing of wounds in this category.	If activity is limited, refer for home services and/or meals-on-wheels.
3. Alteration in elimination	Assess patient's ability to get to toilet. Assess effect of condition on elimination, especially if perianal is involved.	See specific DRG.
4. Alteration in activity and exercise	If skin wound involves lower extremities, the patient may have ambulation difficulties. A consultation with a physical therapist should be done to assess patient's ability to ambulate.	Follow recommendation from physical therapist. Order assistive devices needed prior to discharge.
5. Pain management	Assess patient's level of pain and tolerance of pain medication. Some conditions in this category take a long time to heal, and the patient may need pain control throughout the course.	Explore methods of pain control, including medication, use of warmth and diversional activities.
6. Self-perception, body image disturbance	If the skin wound is visible or will leave scarring, assess the patient's ability to cope with the condition. For patients who are undergoing mastectomy, evaluation of the effect on the body is very important.	During a short-term hospital stay, assessment of this pattern is difficult. If there is any clue that there is a problem, a referral to home nursing should be done. All mastectomy patients should be referred to "Reach for Recovery" from The American Cancer Society.
7. Role-relationship pattern	Assess impact of condition on relationships. If hospitalized patient is responsible for the care of another person in the home, this will have impact on the patient. Assess impact of mastectomy on relationship with the woman's significant other.	See Plan #6 above.

Total Mastectomy for Malignancy – Age > = 70 and/or CC

OPERATIVE PROCEDURE WITH POTENTIAL HOME CARE NEEDS

Total mastectomy

POTENTIAL HOME CARE PROBLEMS	PLAN
1. Health management deficit secondary to age of patient or other illness.	Assess patient's ability to comply with health regime for other illness. If the malignancy is a new diagnosis, this will affect patient's ability to cope with disease; therefore allow patient an opportunity to adjust to diagnosis before beginning teaching.
2. Impaired mobility related to muscle involvement.	If the surgical procedure involved muscles necessary in moving the arm, institute range of motion exercises as soon as possible after surgery. Assess patient's ability to bathe and dress herself and care for the surgical wound.
3. Interruption in role-relationship pattern.	Assess impact of the mastectomy on the patient's socialization. Give the patient information on breast prosthesis. Allow verbalization of impact of surgery on body image. Allow patient to verbalize about diagnosis and prognosis.

REFERRAL INFORMATION

Depending on the patient's living arrangements and availability of primary caregiver, a referral for a home care nurse to monitor disease progress, other disease entity's progress, healing of wound and ability to carry out ADLs is necessary. If the patient was receiving home care services for other disease condition prior to admission, refer for continuation. Refer to American Cancer Society for follow-up support to the patient and for further education of disease process.

Total Mastectomy for Malignancy – Age < 70 w/o CC

OPERATIVE PROCEDURES WITH POTENTIAL HOME CARE NEEDS

See **DRG 257.**

DRG 259

| MDC 09 | RW$ 1.0141 | Surgical | Outlier Cutoff 27 | Mean LOS 7.4 |

Subtotal Mastectomy for Malignancy – Age > = 70 and/or CC

OPERATIVE PROCEDURES WITH POTENTIAL HOME CARE NEEDS

See **DRG 257.**

DETAILS TO CONSIDER

There is no involvement of muscles used to move; therefore there should be no effect on ability to do ADLs.

DRG 260

| MDC 09 | RW$ 0.9325 | Surgical | Outlier Cutoff 26 | Mean LOS 6.4 |

Subtotal Mastectomy for Malignancy – Age < 70

See **DRG 257.**

DRG 261

| MDC 09 | RW$ 0.7329 | Surgical | Outlier Cutoff 19 | Mean LOS 4.8 |

Breast Procedures for Nonmalignancies Except Biopsy and Local Excision

OPERATIVE PROCEDURES WITH POTENTIAL HOME CARE NEEDS

Reduction mammoplasty
Augmentation mammoplasty
Mammoplasty

DETAILS TO CONSIDER

These procedures are done on an elective basis; therefore long-term needs are planned for prior to hospitalization. Patient teaching should include signs and symptoms of infection.

MDC 09   RW$ 0.4617   Surgical   Outlier Cutoff 10   Mean LOS 3.0

Breast Biopsy and Local Excision for Nonmalignancy

OPERATIVE PROCEDURES WITH POTENTIAL HOME CARE NEEDS

Breast biopsy
Local excision of lesion

DETAILS TO CONSIDER

The long-term needs will depend on the biopsy results. If there is a malignancy, the patient will be readmitted under another DRG code in this MDC.

MDC 09   RW$ 2.4737   Surgical   Outlier Cutoff 41   Mean LOS 21.3

Skin Grafts for Skin Ulcer or Cellulitis – Age $>= 70$ and/or CC

OPERATIVE PROCEDURES WITH POTENTIAL HOME CARE NEEDS

Skin graft for cellulitis, any site
Decubitus ulcer
Chronic skin ulcer

DETAILS TO CONSIDER

These are usually long-term home care problems for patients in this group.

POTENTIAL HOME CARE PROBLEMS	PLAN
1. Health management problem secondary to wound management.	Develop a procedure for care of the wound and teach patient and caregiver the procedure. Include the donor site also.
2. Interruption in activity and exercise.	Determine patient's ability to ambulate to carry out activities of daily living (ADLs). The location of the lesion will have a direct effect on the patient's ability to do the ADLs.
3. Alteration in nutrition.	Interview patient for actual dietary intake prior to admission, and actual method of grocery shopping and meal preparation.

REFERRAL INFORMATION

Refer to a home care agency for daily wound care and inspection, teaching of family members. After reviewing the procedure, assist the patient and family in procuring necessary supplies. Assess the need for a hospital bed, if the patient is confined to bed, to assist in frequent position changes. Refer to meals-on-wheels for patients needing help with diet. Determine need for assistive devices for ambulating or toileting.

DRG 264

MDC 09	RW$ 2.2031	Surgical	Outlier Cutoff 38	Mean LOS 18.2

Skin Grafts for Skin Ulcer or Cellulitis – Age < 70 w/o CC

See **DRG 263.**

DRG 265

MDC 09	RW$ 1.4959	Surgical	Outlier Cutoff 29	Mean LOS 8.6

Skin Grafts, Except for Skin Ulcer or Cellulitis with CC

OPERATIVE PROCEDURES WITH POTENTIAL HOME CARE NEEDS

Wound debridement
Skin grafts

DETAILS TO CONSIDER

The comorbidity or complication will have an effect on this DRG, especially if it involves diabetes or peripheral vascular disease.

See **DRG 263.**

DRG 266

MDC 09	RW$ 0.9485	Surgical	Outlier Cutoff 26	Mean LOS 5.9

Skin Grafts Except for Skin Ulcer or Cellulitis w/o CC

See **DRG 263.**

| MDC 09 | RW$ 0.6113 | Surgical | Outlier Cutoff 18 | Mean LOS 5.0 |

Perianal and Pilonidal Procedures

OPERATIVE PROCEDURES WITH POTENTIAL HOME CARE NEEDS

Incision of perianal fistula
Anal fistulotomy
Excision of pilonidal cyst

DETAILS TO CONSIDER

The patient can usually manage self-care following these procedures.

POTENTIAL HOME CARE PROBLEMS	PLAN
1. Health management deficit secondary to location of incision.	Assess patient's ability to see and care for wound. Instruct patient and caregiver in plan of care.
2. Alteration in elimination.	Establish bowel routine, including physician — prescribed stool softeners and dietary changes. Instruct patient in hygiene measures to be taken after bowel movements.

REFERRAL INFORMATION

Patients usually can manage self-care. There may be a need for sitz baths. If so, assess patient's ability to manage procedure safely. If the patient needs assistance refer to home care agency for evaluation. Assist patient in procuring dressings or other supplies needed for wound care.

| MDC 09 | RW$ 0.5388 | Surgical | Outlier Cutoff 15 | Mean LOS 3.0 |

Skin, Subcutaneous Tissue and Breast Plastic Procedures

OPERATIVE PROCEDURES WITH POTENTIAL HOME CARE NEEDS

Eyelid procedures
Ear procedures, inner and outer
Rhinoplasty
Septoplasty
Dermabrasion

DETAILS TO CONSIDER

These are usually done on an elective basis and patients are prepared for home care needs prior to admission.

POTENTIAL HOME CARE PROBLEM	PLAN
Health management deficit secondary to wound care.	Teach patient signs and symptoms of infection and wound care procedures.

DRG 269

MDC 09	RW$ 0.9947	Surgical	Outlier Cutoff 26	Mean LOS 5.7

Other Skin, Subcutaneous Tissue and Breast Operating Procedures – Age > = 70 and/or CC

OPERATIVE PROCEDURES WITH POTENTIAL HOME CARE NEEDS

Lymphatic diagnostic procedures
Bone biopsy

DETAILS TO CONSIDER

Long-term care of the patient will depend on the preadmission status and the outcome of the diagnostic tests.

DRG 270

MDC 09	RW$ 0.8123	Surgical	Outlier Cutoff 25	Mean LOS 4.5

Other Skin, Subcutaneous Tissue and Breast Operating Procedures – Age < 70 w/o CC

See **DRG 269.**

DRG 271

MDC 09	RW$ 1.3802	Medical	Outlier Cutoff 32	Mean LOS 12.1

Skin Ulcers

DIAGNOSES WITH POTENTIAL HOME CARE NEEDS

Decubitus ulcer
Chronic ulcer of the leg
Chronic skin ulcer

DETAILS TO CONSIDER

Even though there is no operative procedure on this admission, the postdischarge course is usually similar to those in **DRG 263.**

MDC 09   **RW$ 0.8620**   **Medical**   **Outlier Cutoff 28**   **Mean LOS 7.8**

Major Skin Disorders – Age > = 70 and/or CC

DIAGNOSES WITH POTENTIAL HOME CARE NEEDS

Erythema nodosum
Herpes zoster
Malignant melanoma
Lupus erythematosus
Psoriasis

DETAILS TO CONSIDER

Some of the diagnoses in this group carry poor prognosis in morbidity and mortality and are chronic conditions. Patient is older than 70 and has a comorbidity or complication.

POTENTIAL HOME CARE PROBLEMS

1. Health care deficit secondary to unpredictable disease process and prognosis.

PLAN

Instruct patient in signs and symptoms of complication of each disease. Teach care of skin lesions following doctor's plan of care. If disease process has poor prognosis, home care needs will be greater and will depend on the clinical manifestation of the disease. Refer to DRG's covering the other diagnoses.

2. Alteration in socialization secondary to change in appearance.

Depending on the visibility of lesions the patient may experience social isolation. If the patient gives evidence of social withdrawal or other clues to isolation, counseling is indicated.

REFERRAL INFORMATION

If clinical symptoms appear, such as joint pain or cardiac or nervous system involvement, a referral to a home health agency is indicated. For the patient with lupus erythematosus a referral to a local support group may be indicated.

MDC 09   **RW$ 0.8286**   **Medical**   **Outlier Cutoff 27**   **Mean LOS 7.3**

Major Skin Disorders – Age < 70 w/o CC

See **DRG 272.**

DRG 274

MDC 09	RW$ 1.0108	Medical	Outlier Cutoff 28	Mean LOS 7.5

Malignant Breast Disorders – Age > = 70 and/or CC

DIAGNOSIS WITH POTENTIAL HOME CARE PROBLEMS

Malignant breast disorders

DETAILS TO CONSIDER

This admission is medical; therefore the patient will not have surgery. Long-term and home care needs will depend on the type of therapy being planned for patient (e.g. chemotherapy, radiation therapy).

POTENTIAL HOME CARE NEEDS

1. Self-care deficit related to need for transportation to and from treatment center if serial treatment is planned.

See **DRG 257.**

PLAN

Assess patient's and caregiver's ability to travel to treatment site for daily treatments. If the treatment is chemotherapy, home IV infusion may be an option.

REFERRAL INFORMATION

Refer to American Cancer Society for assistance in planning transportation. If the patient is a candidate for home IV chemotherapy, consult with the physician on selection of agency to do the treatment; if the hospital has a home IV therapy program, follow the established protocol. If the patient is having difficulty carrying out activities of daily living, or if the disease has metastasized to brain or bone, a referral to a home health agency is indicated.

DRG 275

MDC 09	RW$ 0.0914	Medical	Outlier Cutoff 26	Mean LOS 6.4

Malignant Breast Disorders – Age < 70 w/o CC

See **DRG 274.**

MDC 09   RW$ 0.6066   **Medical**   **Outlier Cutoff 22**   **Mean LOS 4.2**

Nonmalignant Breast Disorders

DIAGNOSES WITH POTENTIAL HOME CARE NEEDS

Benign mammary dysplasia
Fissure of nipple

DETAILS TO CONSIDER

The patient with this diagnosis can normally manage self-care.

MDC 09   RW$ 0.8863   **Medical**   **Outlier Cutoff 28**   **Mean LOS 8.3**

Cellulitis – Age > = 70 and/or CC

DIAGNOSES WITH POTENTIAL HOME CARE NEEDS

Erysipelas
Lymphangitis
Carbuncle
Onychia
Infected laceration of insect bite
Infected foreign body

POTENTIAL HOME CARE PROBLEM

Self-care deficit secondary to wound management.

PLAN

Assess patient's and caregiver's ability to do the wound care.

REFERRAL INFORMATION

Refer to home health agency for wound management if the affected area cannot easily be seen or reached by the patient. If the patient is to receive a 4–6 week course of IV antibiotics, confer with the physician to determine the possibility of home IV therapy. If the patient is a good candidate, refer to home IV therapy company or to your hospital-based program and follow established protocol.

MDC 09   RW$ 0.8096   **Medical**   **Outlier Cutoff 27**   **Mean LOS 7.2**

Cellulitis – Age 18–69 w/o CC

See **DRG 277.**

DRG 279

MDC 09	RW$ 0.4789	Medical	Outlier Cutoff 13	Mean LOS 4.2

Cellulitis – Age 0–17

See **DRG 277.**

The reader is referred to pediatric texts for more information.

DRG 280

MDC 09	RW$ 0.6201	Medical	Outlier Cutoff 25	Mean LOS 5.4

Trauma to the Skin, Subcutaneous Tissue and Breast – Age > = 70 and/or CC

DIAGNOSES WITH POTENTIAL HOME CARE NEEDS

Open wound, any site
Abrasion
Contusion
Multiple contusions

POTENTIAL HOME CARE PROBLEMS

1. Self-care deficit secondary to open wound management.

2. Potential for future injury.

PLAN

Teach patient and caregiver wound care procedure and signs/symptoms of infection.

Determine cause of accident and discuss accident prevention.

REFERRAL INFORMATION

If there is *any* suspicion that the trauma is the result of physical abuse, a referral to the proper authorities is mandatory. If the wound is in an area that the patient cannot see or reach, or if it impairs the patient's ability to carry out activities of daily living, a referral for home nursing is indicated.

DRG 281

MDC 09	RW$ 0.5377	Medical	Outlier Cutoff 23	Mean LOS 4.2

Trauma to the Skin, Subcutaneous Tissue and Breast – Age 18–69 w/o CC

See **DRG 280.**

MDC 09	RW$ 0.3460	Medical	Outlier Cutoff 9	Mean LOS 2.2

Trauma to the Skin, Subcutaneous Tissue and Breast – Age 0–17

See **DRG 280.**

The reader is referred to pediatric texts for more information.

MDC 09	RW$ 0.6394	Medical	Outlier Cutoff 25	Mean LOS 5.3

Minor Skin Disorders – Age $>= 70$ and/or CC

DIAGNOSES WITH POTENTIAL HOME CARE NEEDS

Plastic surgery
Viral warts
Herpes simplex
Cancer in situ of the skin
Dermatitis
Diseases of the nail
Hair disease
Sweat gland disorder

DETAILS TO CONSIDER

Patients with these diagnoses can usually manage their own care, unless the complication or comorbidity affects their ability to do so.

See DRGs related to comorbidity or complication.

MDC 09	RW$ 0.5971	Medical	Outlier Cutoff 24	Mean LOS 4.4

Minor Skin Disorders – Age < 70 w/o CC

See **DRG 283.**

10 MDC 10
ENDOCRINE, NUTRITIONAL AND METABOLIC DISEASES AND DISORDERS

SURGICAL GROUPINGS (9 DRGs)

Amputations

Adrenal and Pituitary Procedures

Skin Grafts and Wound Debridement

OR Procedures for Obesity

Parathyroid, Thyroid and Thyroglossal Procedures

Other OR Procedures

MEDICAL GROUPINGS (8 DRGs)

Diabetes

Nutritional and Miscellaneous Disorders

Inborn Errors of Metabolism

Endocrine Disorders

MASTER HOME CARE PLANNING GUIDE FOR ENDOCRINE, NUTRITIONAL AND METABOLIC DISEASES AND DISORDERS

Pattern	Assessment Factors	Plan
1. Health management deficit with potential for noncompliance	Previous health care practices with emphasis on past compliance with medical regime. Financial resources information since many diagnoses in this category are chronic and costly medications are required. Are there other complications of the disorder that make self-care more difficult, such as visual impairment or peripheral vascular impairment? What is the health status of the caregiver or significant other?	Interview patient and significant other. Review health history. Initiate discussion of health insurance or financial resources to determine the need for social service intervention.
2. Alteration in nutrition	Thorough assessment of nutritional status necessary in these disorders. Diet therapy may represent a dramatic change in patient's dietary habits. Understanding of prescribed diet and rationale for such. Determine patient/family total dietary needs, preferences, social customs and ability to grocery shop and prepare meals.	Take a thorough nutritional history. Involve clinical dietician. Patient/family history should be taken to help determine learning needs. Assist in planning diet of patient keeping family needs in mind.
3. Alteration in elimination	Digestive process may be impaired with a potential for either temporary or permanent alteration in urinary or bowel elimination problems. Although the gastrointestinal and renal systems are not directly involved, they are affected by some endocrine functions and by nutritional disorders. A detailed history and assessment of these systems may reveal long-term problems that need intervention.	See specific DRG.
4. Activity and exercise: **4a.** activity tolerance	History of patient's tolerance for activity and exercise.	See specific DRG.
4b. mobility impaired	Patient's functional ability to carry out self-care and activities of daily living must be assessed.	

4c. home maintenance management deficit	Assess level of home management deficit as mild, moderate, severe, potential or chronic.	Interview patient/family to determine physical environment of home and financial resources. Instruct regarding home patient care needs. Determine potential home management deficit with consideration for: • specific diagnosis. • severity of illness. • level of care required. • ability and availability of caregiver.
5. Cognitive/perceptual pattern: **5a.** alteration in comfort (pain)	Pain can occur as a result of surgery or as a complication of some chronic diseases. Such pain can limit daily function.	Assess pain threshold. Determine previous coping mechanisms used to deal with pain (medication, diversional activity). Assess effectiveness of analgesics.
5b. knowledge deficit regarding disease process and self-care.	Baseline knowledge — patient's perception of information needed to cope with diagnosis. Assess patient's understanding of need for long-term hormone replacement following some surgeries in this category.	Assess patient's ability and willingness to be involved in self-care. Patient and/or family education regarding self-care needs, disease process.
6. Alteration in self-perception, body image disturbance	Diagnoses with chronic disease can alter self-perception. Surgical procedures can alter body image, especially limb amputation.	Explore patient's feelings related to illness or surgery. Discuss availability of prostheses where applicable. Discuss availability of support groups if needed. See specific DRG.
7. Potential for sexual dysfunction	Some chronic diseases can alter sexual function. Many patients are reluctant to discuss this issue despite the fact that sexual function can be central to their self-image.	If gland involved or disease process will hinder or has hindered sexual function, refer patient for counseling.
8. Coping/stress tolerance pattern	Living with chronic disease can place emotional and financial strain on the individual and/or family due to frequent and prolonged hospitalization. Chronic disease may be responsible for absence from work or may be used by employers as reason for not hiring or dismissing from work situation. Diseases of this system are often negatively affected by stress.	Refer to social service for financial resource assistance.

DRG 285

MDC 10	RW$ 2.8658	Surgical	Outlier Cutoff 44	Mean LOS 24.0

Amputations for Endocrine, Nutritional and Metabolic Disorders

OPERATIVE PROCEDURES WITH POTENTIAL HOME CARE NEEDS

Lower limb amputations

See **DRG 113** (amputation).

See **DRGs 294** and **295** (diabetes).

DETAILS TO CONSIDER

The amputations for this DRG result from complications from the disease; there may be several other complications occurring at the same time.

POTENTIAL HOME CARE PROBLEMS	PLAN
1. Health management deficit related to noncompliance.	Assess patient's understanding of medical care for the original diagnosis. Stress importance of follow-up to prevent further complications.
2. Alteration in activity and exercise pattern.	Since patient has an amputation, there will be a change in activity. The dietary requirements may change; thus a modification of the diet will be needed.
3. Alteration in self-concept secondary to complication of amputation.	The patient may need counseling and should be referred to a rehabilitation program.

REFERRAL INFORMATION

The patient's referral needs will depend on the ability to transfer or ambulate, the strength of the caregiver and his/her ability to help the patient move. It will also depend on the status of the prosthetic device. This DRG has a relatively long length of stay, and the patient should be relatively independent in activities of daily living at the time of discharge. Referrals for adaptive equipment in the home and for the patient's care need to be made. If the underlying metabolic condition needs to be monitored, a referral for follow-up care should be made.

DRG 286

MDC 10	RW$ 2.8952	Surgical	Outlier Cutoff 36	Mean LOS 16.1

Adrenal and Pituitary Procedures

OPERATIVE PROCEDURES WITH POTENTIAL HOME CARE NEEDS

Adrenalectomy, unilateral and bilateral
Transphenoid pituitary operations
Pineal operations

DETAILS TO CONSIDER

In some of these procedures the most important long-term need is for hormone replacement therapy. Also, the medical reason for the procedure will need to be evaluated. For example, if the procedure is done for palliation of a malignancy, or because of a malignancy, many other follow-up plans will need to be addressed.

POTENTIAL HOME CARE PROBLEM	PLAN
Alteration in self-care.	Determine patient's level of understanding of medical plan for follow-up care, especially for replacement therapy.

REFERRAL INFORMATION

Patient may need referral for a home care nurse to monitor ability to self-administer hormone replacement and monitor progression of disease. If procedure was done for a malignancy, referral to a hospice program is indicated.

DRG 287

MDC 10	RW$ 2.8143	Surgical	Outlier Cutoff 43	Mean LOS 22.8

Skin Grafts and Wound Debridement for Endocrine, Nutritional and Metabolic Disorders

OPERATIVE PROCEDURES WITH POTENTIAL HOME CARE NEEDS

Skin grafts and wound debridement for endocrine, nutritional and metabolic disorders

See **DRGs 263** and **264, 294** and **295.**

DETAILS TO CONSIDER

Most of the procedures in this group result from diabetic complications.

POTENTIAL HOME CARE PROBLEM	PLAN
Self-care deficit secondary to wound care.	Assess patient's/caregiver's ability to care for wound. Give detailed written instructions to the patient.

REFERRAL INFORMATION

Refer to a home care nurse for wound care follow-up procedure set up in the home. Refer patient to a source to buy supplies and have available on the day of discharge. Include in the referral to the home care nurse information on the patient's diagnosis, medical regime and compliance.

DRG 288

MDC 10	RW$ 1.5695	Surgical	Outlier Cutoff 24	Mean LOS 10.0

Operating Room Procedures for Obesity

OPERATIVE PROCEDURES WITH POTENTIAL HOME CARE NEEDS

Gastric bypass
Intestinal anastomosis

DETAILS TO CONSIDER

These procedures are done on younger people who are relatively stable medically. This is an elective procedure; therefore plans for follow-up should be made prior to admission.

POTENTIAL HOME CARE PROBLEMS	PLAN
1. Alteration in activity/exercise.	Patient should be instructed in exercise program to enhance muscle tone and cardiac status.
2. Alteration in self-perception.	Allow patient to verbalize anticipated changes in lifestyle.

REFERRAL INFORMATION

Patient's health status should be stable and patient should only need medical follow-up.

DRG 289

MDC 10	RW$ 1.3736	Surgical	Outlier Cutoff 28	Mean LOS 8.3

Parathyroid Procedures

OPERATIVE PROCEDURES WITH POTENTIAL HOME CARE NEEDS

Parathyroidectomy

DETAILS TO CONSIDER

The parathyroid hormones affect the bone, kidney and gastrointestinal tract; therefore the needs of the patient will depend on what the effect of the disease condition has been on these three sites. There may also be other disease conditions occurring at the same time.

MDC 10	RW$ 0.8549	Surgical	Outlier Cutoff 17	Mean LOS 6.0

Thyroid Procedures

OPERATIVE PROCEDURES WITH POTENTIAL HOME CARE NEEDS

Partial thyroidectomy
Total thyroidectomy

DETAILS TO CONSIDER

The patient may need thyroid hormone replacement therapy. In partial thyroidectomy the patient will need to have close medical follow-up to determine adequacy of thyroid hormone.

MDC 10	RW$ 0.4909	Surgical	Outlier Cutoff 8	Mean LOS 2.9

Thyroglossal Procedures

OPERATIVE PROCEDURES WITH POTENTIAL HOME CARE NEEDS

Thyroglossal duct excision

DETAILS TO CONSIDER

This condition is due to a developmental defect in which a cyst forms on the thyroglossal duct. The excision of the cyst is usually done as an inpatient because of the extent of the procedure. Follow-up care is usually accomplished in the physician's office.

MDC 10	RW$ 2.0307	Surgical	Outlier Cutoff 31	Mean LOS 10.8

Other Endocrine, Nutritional and Metabolic Operating Room Procedures – Age > = 70 and/or CC

OPERATIVE PROCEDURES WITH POTENTIAL HOME CARE NEEDS

Thymectomy
Insert testicular prosthesis

DETAILS TO CONSIDER

Home care and long-term needs will be related to the procedure and underlying diagnosis.

DRG 293

| MDC 10 | RW$ 1.4951 | Surgical | Outlier Cutoff 28 | Mean LOS 8.0 |

Other Endocrine, Nutritional and Metabolic Operating Room Procedures – Age < 70 w/o CC

See **DRG 292.**

DRG 294

| MDC 10 | RW$ 0.8087 | Medical | Outlier Cutoff 28 | Mean LOS 7.7 |

Diabetes – Age > = 36

DIAGNOSTIC PROCEDURES WITH POTENTIAL HOME CARE NEEDS

Diabetes, uncomplicated
Diabetes, coma
Diabetes, hyperosmolar coma

DETAILS TO CONSIDER

Patient's understanding of disease process and proposed plan of care will be crucial to his/her ability to cope with diabetes. Fear and anxiety may affect acceptance of diagnosis. Patients with limited intelligence, impaired vision or other specific problems may require follow-up in the home to assess compliance with plan. Concomitant illnesses can lead to the development of coma.

POTENTIAL HOME CARE PROBLEMS

1. Health management deficit potential related to need for long-term medical follow-up.

2. Alleviation in nutrition related to impaired glucose metabolism. Dietary noncompliance can lead to hyperglycemia, diabetic ketoacidosis, or hyperosmolar coma.

3. Potential for alteration in bowel or bladder function related to autonomic neuropathy.

PLAN

Assess patient's understanding of need for medical follow-up and rationale for proposed treatment regimen. Assess degree to which patient is limited in self-care ability by complications of diabetes (i.e. visual, sensory). Need to instruct patient about appropriate diet, avoidance of concentrated sweets, and balance in carbohydrates, protein and fat. Involve diet team as indicated.

Assess understanding of and compliance with prescribed diet. Teaching should involve family members or significant others involved in food preparation. Determine patient's dietary needs based on type of diabetes and mode of treatment.

Educate patient regarding possibility of complications (i.e. neurogenic bladder, diabetic diarrhea, gastroparesis) and appropriate treatment, Provide emotional support.

4. Activity and exercise essential to long-term control of diabetes. Exercise can lower blood sugar levels, increasing risk of hypoglycemia.

Encourage daily exercise. Suggest exercise plans according to patient's level of health and mobility. Stress importance of exercise in maintaining control of blood sugar. Teach patient regarding possible need for extra carbohydrates prior to exercise to prevent hypoglycemia.

5. Knowledge deficit regarding self-care activities and disease process.

Determine baseline understanding about disease and prescribed treatment. Assess patient's comprehension of specific activities by requesting a return demonstration of technique. If education is insufficient, arrange for continued teaching as outpatient.

6. Altered self-perception related to chronic disease state.

Emotional support for patient and family. Identify community diabetes support groups.

7. Sexual dysfunction related to diabetic neuropathy.

Assess degree to which patient is affected by sexual dysfunction. Patient education and sexual counseling is indicated.

8. Ineffective coping related to chronic disease state.

Assess degree to which diabetic control is affected by stress. Examine cause of stress with patient and explore possible methods of coping. Educate patient and family about the negative effect of stress on diabetes control. Counseling as indicated.

REFERRAL INFORMATION

Background information — health history, onset of diabetes, complications, and family situation, should be communicated to the home care nurse. History of current hospitalization including complications. Diabetes education received in hospital including patient's ability to perform self-care tasks. Include need for assist devices (i.e. magnifying glass). Include type of equipment/methods used in education (i.e. urine test method, syringe brand). Include prescribed diet and meal pattern.

Refer to Meals-on-Wheels program or adult day-care program that includes prescribed diet plan for patients who may otherwise have difficulty getting meals.

DRG 295

MDC 10	RW$ 0.7457	Surgical	Outlier Cutoff 26	Mean LOS 5.6

Diabetes – Age 0–35

DIAGNOSTIC PROCEDURES WITH POTENTIAL HOME CARE NEEDS

Diabetes, uncomplicated
Diabetes, coma
Diabetes, hyperosmolar coma

DETAILS TO CONSIDER

Same as **DRG 294.**

For children and adolescents, responsibility of care will rest with the parent. The age at which a child accepts responsibility for self-care is very individualized.

Young people tend to have Type I diabetes, a more brittle and severe form of the disease. People with Type I diabetes are more prone to diabetic ketoacidosis (diabetic coma), especially in relation to illness.

Young women of child-bearing age should be informed of the importance of close medical follow-up prior to and during pregnancy, because of the increased risk of complications, including ketoacidosis in the mother.

POTENTIAL HOME CARE PROBLEMS

Same as **DRG 294.**

1. Alteration in nutrition related to growth and maturation.

2. Denial of diagnosis and necessary treatment can lead to uncontrolled diabetes.

PLAN

Educate patient and family regarding changing caloric needs in relation to growth and maturation.

Counseling as indicated. Encourage parents to allow increased self-care and independence based on child's readiness.

REFERRAL INFORMATION

Contact with school nurse following initial diagnosis in children or in relation to repeated episodes of uncontrolled diabetes. Same as **DRG 294.**

DRG 296

MDC 10	RW$ 0.8979	Medical	Outlier Cutoff 27	Mean LOS 7.3

Nutritional and Miscellaneous Disorders – Age > = 70 and/or CC

DIAGNOSTIC PROCEDURES WITH POTENTIAL HOME CARE NEEDS

Hypoglycemia
Kwashiorkor
Malnutrition
Nutrition deficiency
Acidosis/alkalosis
Electrolyte/fluid imbalance
Anorexia

DETAILS TO CONSIDER

Conditions in this group are long-term, and close medical follow-up is necessary. The approach to care will depend on the cause of the problem.

POTENTIAL HOME CARE PROBLEMS

1. Health care deficit related to long-term nature of the diagnosis.

PLAN

Depending on the cause of the problem, instruct patient in expected course of treatment. In all cases, modification of dietary intake will be necessary. The patient and significant other may need counseling to help bring about changes in behavior to improve self-care. Since eating is a social interaction, the whole family may need to be involved.

2. Alteration in nutrition.

Assess patient's nutritional needs and plan nutritional therapy. Choices include oral supplements; tube feedings either by nasogastric route, gastrostomy or other tube into the digestive system; or total parenteral nutrition. Assess the patient's ability to do own therapy in the home. Assess availability of caregiver on a 24-hour basis. Refer to total parenteral nutrition information to develop a teaching plan for the patient. Include teaching of the central line catheter that is the access site for solution infusion.

3. Alteration in elimination.

Teach patient differences to expect in bowel habits dependent on type of nutritional therapy planned. Instruct patient and caregiver in signs and symptoms of impaction and in symptoms of volume depletion and electrolyte imbalance that can result from diarrhea.

4. Changes in activity/exercise.

Instruct patient in need for exercise to establish muscle tone. Instruct patient to gradually increase exercise.

5. Alteration in role-relationship.

Assess effect of patient's illness on relationship and assess psychological impact on patient and family. If malnutrition appears to be from neglect, assess relationships and plan for follow-up.

REFERRAL INFORMATION

Third-party payor (insurance) information should be obtained when making plans for therapy. Total parenteral nutrition is a very expensive and somewhat complicated form of therapy and is reimbursable only under strict conditions. This information must be available during the planning stage.

If the patient receives nutritional feeding through a tube, utilizing a feeding pump, a referral to a home therapy company should be made. Delivering of supplies such as feeding pump, bags, connection tubing, syringes for flushing the line and the feeding and teaching of the patient in the home are services the patient will need. A referral to a home health agency for skilled nursing care should be made, especially if the patient has a gastrostomy tube or any ostomy-type tube.

Medications for patients with feeding tubes should be ordered in liquid form to allow for ease in giving. A feeding tube for long-term therapy has a small diameter and crushed pills can plug the tube, necessitating reinsertion. Note: If the malnutrition appears to be from neglect, contact social services for further investigation. In some states this is mandatory.

DRG 297

MDC 10	RW$ 0.7923	Medical	Outlier Cutoff 26	Mean LOS 6.0

Nutritional and Miscellaneous Metabolic Disorders
Age 18–69 w/o CC

DIAGNOSTIC PROCEDURES WITH POTENTIAL HOME CARE NEEDS

Same as **DRG 296** plus: lack of normal physiological development.

DRG 298

MDC 10 | **RW$ 0.7538** | **Medical** | **Outlier Cutoff 25** | **Mean LOS 5.4**

Nutritional and Miscellaneous Metabolic Disorders – Age 0–17

DIAGNOSTIC PROCEDURES WITH POTENTIAL HOME CARE NEEDS

Same as **DRG 297** plus: feeding problems.

DETAILS TO CONSIDER

See **DRG 296.**

The young child who has a feeding problem or any nutritional or metabolic diagnosis will need long-term care. Refer to pediatric references for additional information.

DRG 299

MDC 10 | **RW$ 0.9407** | **Medical** | **Outlier Cutoff 27** | **Mean LOS 6.8**

Inborn Errors of Metabolism

DIAGNOSTIC PROCEDURES WITH POTENTIAL HOME CARE NEEDS

Phenylketonuria (PKU)
Lipoprotein deficiencies
Galactosemia
Hyperlipidemia

DETAILS TO CONSIDER

For these diagnoses which are made in the pediatric patient, check pediatric references for further information.

POTENTIAL HOME CARE PROBLEM

Health management deficit secondary to change in life-style.

PLAN

Instruct patient in dietary changes, medications, signs and symptoms of conditions which can result from metabolic condition.

Endocrine Disorders – Age > = 70 and/or CC

DIAGNOSTIC PROCEDURES WITH POTENTIAL HOME CARE NEEDS

Thyroid disorders
Parathyroid disorders
Pituitary disorders
Pancreatic disorders
Adrenal disorders
Sexual development abnormality

DETAILS TO CONSIDER

The follow-up care for patients in this group will depend on the primary cause for the disorder. For example, the cause can be an inflammation, a primary malignancy or a metastatic disease. The normal function of the hormone, the effect of hyperfunction or hypofunction on other body systems and the effect of a diseased gland on organs in close proximity must be evaluated before long-term follow-up can be planned. If any of the above leaves the patient in a compromised condition, a referral for appropriate follow-up should be made.

DRG 301   DRG 301

MDC 10   RW$ 0.8143   Medical   Outlier Cutoff 26   Mean LOS 6.4

Endocrine Disorders – Age < 70 w/o CC

Same as **DRG 300**.

11

MDC 11
DISEASES AND DISORDERS
OF THE KIDNEY AND URINARY TRACT

SURGICAL GROUPINGS (14 DRGs)

Kidney Transplant

Kidney, Ureter and Major Bladder Procedures

Prostatectomy

Minor Bladder Procedures

Urethral and Transurethral Procedures

MEDICAL GROUPINGS (18 DRGs)

Renal Failure with and w/o Dialysis

Kidney and Urinary Tract Neoplasms and Infections

Urinary Stones

Urethral Stricture

MASTER HOME CARE PLANNING GUIDE
FOR CONDITIONS AFFECTING THE KIDNEY AND URINARY TRACT

Pattern	Assessment Factors	Plan
1. Health perception; health management	Is this illness event an acute manifestation of a chronic condition or an isolated acute illness?	See specific DRG.
	What was the patient's prehospitalization level of functioning?	Interview the patient and significant other.
	How does the patient perceive his/her illness in relation to the ability to function at prehospitalization level?	Interview the patient and caregiver.
	What is the patient's prognosis? Does the patient know and understand the prognosis?	Refer to medical record, primary physician, patient and family.
	NOTE: Many illnesses in this MDC significantly alter previous level of functioning.	Involve social services, chaplain, oncology clinician as appropriate to meet patient's needs.
	Does the potential for noncompliance to the medical regimen exist?	See specific DRG and referral information.
	Is there increased potential for complications involving other organs and systems due to renal disease?	See specific DRG.
2. Alteration in nutrition	What was the nutritional status of the patient prior to present illness?	Interview patient and family.
	What is patient's present state of nutrition?	Assess nutritional parameters: height/weight ratio, serum albumin transfusions, % weight loss or gain from usual.
	What cultural influences affect patient's perception of nutrition and dietary habits?	See specific DRG.
	What effect does present illness have on the need to alter usual dietary patterns?	NOTE: Medical management of chronic renal failure involves dietary restrictions.
	Will dietary changes place a financial burden on patient and family?	Involve social services.
	What effect do illness, medications, mental and emotional status have on patient's appetite and gastrointestinal functioning?	See specific DRG. Review caloric counts. Review weight loss/gain patterns. Assess for occult GI bleeding by hematesting stools.
	NOTE: Magnesium-containing laxatives or antacids are contraindicated for patients with renal disease due to decreased ability of kidney to filter magnesium, creating hypermagnesemia resulting in CNS depression and irritability.	Interview patient to assess need for laxatives, enemas, or stool softeners. Interview patient and family and involve person who prepares the meals in dietary teaching. Consult with dietician.

	What effect will patient's dietary regime have on other family members and person responsible for meal preparation?	
3. Alteration in elimination (urine)	Does the patient have lingering S/S of urinary dysfunction at time of discharge?	Review medical record. Interview the patient to elicit his/her perception of urinary function. See specific DRG.
	Does the patient have a urinary diversion such as a cystostomy, ileal conduit?	See specific DRG.
	Does the patient need assistance in managing urinary collection appliance?	Involve ostomy clinician.
	Does the patient depend on intermittent catheterization or permanent indwelling catheter for urinary discharge?	See specific DRG.
	Is the patient or significant other able to perform procedures independently?	Involve an ostomy therapist.
	Are there special equipment needs for home management of urinary diversion and/or drainage?	See specific DRG. Inform patient and family how and where to obtain essential supplies. Ensure that the patient has enough supplies at time of discharge to handle immediate needs.
	Will equipment needs create a financial burden to patient/family?	Involve social services. Investigate community services for support.
	Are there specific S/S of renal dysfunction that the patient must monitor after discharge?	See specific DRG. Ensure that patient and family teaching is adequate — obtain feedback.
3a. (stool)	Does the patient have the potential for GI complications due to illness?	See specific DRG.
	What is the patient's normal bowel routine and has present illness altered this?	Interview patient.
	Does the medication prescribed for patient's illness have the potential to alter bowel elimination patterns?	Refer to 'Alteration in Nutrition'. See specific DRG. Review list of medications. Assess patient for S/S of bowel dysfunction.
4. Activity and exercise	Is nature of illness self-limiting in regard to deficit in level of activity, or will there be chronic disability with decreasing activity tolerance over time?	See specific DRG.
	Is there a potential for lethargy, muscle wasting and decreased exercise tolerance due to prescribed medications?	See specific DRG. Ensure patient education of these effects and method to combat disabilities. Obtain patient feedback.

Does the potential for renal osteodystrophy exist? NOTE: Decalcification of bones is a frequent complication of renal disease due to impaired metabolism of vitamin D resulting in decreased absorption of calcium via the gut, as well as impaired renal filtration of phosphorus resulting in hypocalcemia.	See specific DRG.
Does patient need assistive devices for safe ambulation, transfer activities, or is patient wheelchair-dependent or bedridden?	Instruct and assist patient and family in the procurement and safe use of necessary equipment and installation of safety bars and rails. Involve physical therapist.
Does the patient require a specific physical therapy regimen?	See specific DRG. Involve physical therapist in the arrangements for patient after discharge.

5. Cognitive — perceptual deficit.

Do the consequences of the physical illness result in decrease in ability to concentrate, impaired judgment and intellectual functioning and ability to make sound decisions?	See specific DRG.
Is the patient able to function safely in self-care routines at the level performed prior to hospitalization?	Interview patient and family.
Does medication prescribed for illness or pain control impair patient's ability to function at a safe level for independence.	Assess need for supervision and supportive care by observing patient while under influence of medications.

6. Alteration in self-perception and self-concept

Has the patient experienced an alteration in physical appearance due to specific illness and/or its medical management?	See specific DRG.
What effect has the alteration in physical appearances had on the patient's body image?	Discuss with patient feelings regarding physical changes. Offer support and concrete suggestions on ways to combat or counteract unacceptable effects, i.e., concealment of ostomy appliance, weight control, exercise program, bleaching or removal of excess facial/body hair. See specific DRG.
Has the illness created dependency needs in a formerly independent person? NOTE: Home dialysis patients depend on a partner for management of dialysis routines.	Assess the effects of patient's loss of contact and independence on emotional status and willingness to accept help from others. Assess the ability of the patient's family to accept patient's dependency needs. Involve social service for counseling.

234

7. Alteration in role-relationship	Has the patient experienced change in normal role patterns due to illness, such as parenting role, breadwinner role, friendship role, sexual role and marital role?	Involve social service for ongoing support. Assess effect of role changes on patient's financial status, family and social relationships. Assess ability of family/significant other to cope and adapt to role changes.
	What effect has patient's illness had on his/her sense of self-worth?	Encourage patient to verbalize concerns and emphasize the positive capabilities and contributions that the patient can make.
8. Alteration in sexuality and reproduction	Has the patient experienced sexual dysfunction, impotence, decreased libido due to illness or effects of medications? NOTE: Many antihypertensive medications used in the treatment of renal disease cause sexual dysfunction. Reduction in dosage or change of medication may be necessary to counteract these effects.	Counsel the patient that effects are usually temporary and often can be reversed. Encourage the patient to verbalize fears.
	Has the patient expressed a diminished self-image as a sexual being due to physical changes resulting from illness and/or surgery?	Involve social services for counseling.
	Has the illness created sterility/infertility? Due to the risk of genetic transmission of certain renal diseases (polycystic renal disease), has the patient been advised to refrain from having children?	See specific DRG.
	Will pregnancy aggravate the mother's renal disease or impose a risk on the developing fetus?	Involve social service for counseling.
9. Alteration in ability to cope	Has the patient exhibited changes in normal behavior pattern?	Involve social services for counseling patient and caregiver.
	Assess for irritability, tearfulness, depression, insomnia, loss of appetite, apathy and demanding behavior. NOTE: Chronic illness creates stress and anxieties that may overwhelm patient's normal coping mechanism.	Provide patient with factual information so that he/she will not aggravate stress because of ungrounded fears. Verbalize to patient realistic expectations of the prognosis.
10. Spirituality	Has the patient expressed the need for spiritual counseling? NOTE: Patient may view illness as a punishment for past wrongdoing.	Involve the patient's personal minister and/or chaplain to offer spiritual guidance to the patient and family. NOTE: Patient may receive comfort from this intervention, particularly when offered prior to surgery or at decision-making times.

DRG 302

Kidney Transplant

OPERATIVE PROCEDURE WITH POTENTIAL HOME CARE NEEDS

Kidney transplant

DETAILS TO CONSIDER

Prognoses and degree of complications are affected by the amount of immunosuppression required to prevent rejection of the transplanted kidney. Recipients of living related donor kidneys now experience a greater than 90% graft survival; moreover, due to more compatible tissue typing, they require less immunosuppression than cadaver kidney transplants. These patients currently enjoy a 70% graft survival.

Age and other compromising conditions associated with chronic renal failure also affect the outcome of renal transplantation.

POTENTIAL HOME CARE PROBLEMS

PLAN

1. Health management deficit related to need for long-term medical management and need to adhere to medication regimen to achieve graft survival.

Patient teaching should be initiated early in the course of hospitalization, and adequate feedback to assess the patient's understanding should be obtained. Written instructions should be given to the patient prior to discharge, including medications, diet, activity level, exercise program, medical follow-up schedule, specimen collection routines, and signs and symptoms suggesting rejection or other complications. Involve social services to assist patient in managing financial problems related to cost of medications and other expenses.

2. Nutrition related to dietary restrictions. NOTE: With successful transplantation, most dietary restrictions imposed due to chronic renal failure are removed. Sodium restriction is often continued, as well as a diet compatible with body weight goals. Steroid medications given to prevent rejection frequently cause an increase in appetite, which may lead to obesity if not controlled. Successful transplantation allows the patient to enjoy many foods previously forbidden.

Diet instruction and assessment of patient's understanding through independent menu situation should be accomplished prior to discharge.

3. Elimination (stool) related to side effects of medication regimen. NOTE: many antacids prescribed for the transplant recipient alter normal bowel habits, most frequently resulting in constipation. An untoward complication of steroid administration is GI irritation, manifesting as black/tarry stools.

Instruct patient to notify physician if a change in color, consistency and frequency of bowel movements is experienced.

Elimination (urine) related to signs of kidney rejection, infection or other complications.

Instruct patient to report any change in volume, hematuria frequency, urgency, or burning on urination.

4. Activity and exercise related to effects of medications and placement of graft. NOTE: chronic steroid administration causes muscle wasting, particularly in the legs and arms. Antihypertensive drugs often cause lethargy. The transplanted graft is surgically placed in the anterior pelvis iliac fossa, which is a less protected environment than the native renal location.

Instruct patient to adhere to established exercise program. Stair climbing and walking are preferred exercises. Advise patient to avoid contact sports and activities that have the potential to injure the transplanted kidney.

5. Self-perception/self-concept related to changes in physical appearance. NOTE: steroid medications cause a cushingoid appearance which often creates the need for a major psychological adjustment.

Advise patient that these side effects will decrease if/when the dosage is lowered. Offer suggestions on ways to improve appearance such as weight control, exercise program and application of cosmetics.

6. Role-relationship related to improved state of health resulting from successful transplantation. NOTE: discarding the sick role requires major role adjustments for patient and family members.

Counsel patient and family that a gradual return to pre-illness roles with minor adjustments is usually an obtainable goal.

7. Sexuality — reproduction related to medications and stress of pregnancy. NOTE: antihypertensive medications sometimes cause impotence and decreased libido.

Instruct patient that side effects that bear on sexuality caused by some medications can be reduced with dosage and/or medication adjustment. Female patients should be advised that they may resume menstruation with improved renal function. Pregnancy is discouraged due to the added burden of the developing fetus, as well as for the untoward effects of the prescribed medications on the fetus.

8. Value-belief pattern related to donor source. NOTE: the transplant recipient may have psychological problems in accepting the donor kidney. NOTE: the patient may fantasize that he/she is taking on characteristics of the donor. This is particularly a problem if the donor is from the opposite sex. The recipient may feel guilty of depriving the living-related donor of his/her second kidney. The recipient may have religious or cultural beliefs that interfere with the incorporation of the transplanted organ.

Offer appropriate psychological and emotional support to the patient and family. Involve the social worker or psychiatrist for counseling as indicated by the patient's behavior.

REFERRAL INFORMATION

The need for referral depends on the degree of patient's understanding and compliance with the medical management protocol. Medication management is the primary reason for most referrals. Referral information should include institution's patient teaching protocols, patient's compliance history, and patient's physical psychological and emotional strengths and limitations.

DRG 303

MDC 11   RW$ 2.5397   Surgical   Outlier Cutoff 36   Mean LOS 16.2

Kidney, Ureter and Major Bladder Procedure for Neoplasm

Principal diagnoses are malignant neoplasm of the bladder, kidney, ureter or urethra.

OPERATIVE PROCEDURES WITH POTENTIAL HOME CARE NEEDS

Nephrectomy
Ureterectomy
Radical or total cystectomy

DETAILS TO CONSIDER

Prognosis depends on ability to eradicate neoplasm and prevent or treat distant metastasis. Loss of one kidney does not significantly affect renal function. Normal filtering and elimination of wastes are achievable with a single kidney. Urinary diversion procedures often result in an ostomy, necessitating major adjustments in elimination habits.

POTENTIAL HOME CARE PROBLEMS

PLAN

1. Health management deficit related to prognosis, chronicity of illness and potential for complications.

Involve social service and oncology clinician for counseling. Instruct patient that long-term medical follow-up is essential to maintain state of health.

2. Alteration in nutrition related to amount of renal function remaining. NOTE: no restrictions may be needed if adequate renal function is present. With impaired renal function, protein, sodium, potassium and fluid volume restrictions may be necessary.

Discharge diet instructions should be given to patient and family, with feedback obtained of their level of understanding. Involve the dietician.

3. Alteration in elimination of urine related to the amount of renal function remaining, neurogenic bladder, and/or presence of diversionary stoma, such as an ileoconduit.

Instruct patient to notify physician of any change in urine color, odor, volume, hematuria or signs of infection, including cloudy urine, urgency and frequency. Involve enterostomal therapist for assistance in patient acceptance and management of urostomy. Instruct patient and/or significant other on management of urostomy and where to obtain supplies and equipment. Involve social service for assistance in managing finances if needed. Instruct patient in self-catheterization technique if required to treat neurogenic bladder.

4. Self-perception/self-concept deficit related to malignant disease and/or alteration in body image.

Encourage patient to verbalize concerns, emotions and fears. Involve social service for counseling.

5. Role-relationship related to potential loss of independence as a result of terminal process. NOTE: patient may experience feelings of hopelessness and uselessness with diminishing ability to perform self-care routines.

Allow patient to remain in control and make all decisions that they are capable of making. Offer choices when able and follow patient's wishes when possible.

6. Sexuality — reproduction deficit related to specific disease process and result of surgical procedure.

Instruct patient on ability or lack of ability to reproduce or participate in sexual intercourse. Offer sexual counseling when indicated.

7. Value — belief pattern related to illness, prognosis, death and dying.

Involve social service and spiritual leader for counseling. Encourage patient to verbalize concerns and fears. Anticipate stages of death and dying and counsel family in progression.

REFERRAL INFORMATION

Referral should include: level of independence in care of urinary diversion, neurogenic bladder or incontinence; what supplies and equipment are being used for urostomy or self-catheterization and where they may be obtained; patient's prognosis and understanding and acceptance of illness; patient's ability to perform activities of daily living. Durable medical equipment requirements will depend on patient's condition.

DRG 304

| MDC 11 | RW$ 1.7952 | Surgical | Outlier Cutoff 33 | Mean LOS 12.8 |

Kidney, Ureter and Major Bladder Procedure for Nonmalignancy – Age > = 70 and/or CC

OPERATIVE PROCEDURES WITH POTENTIAL HOME CARE NEEDS

Rejected kidney nephrectomy
Nephrostomy
Cutaneous ileoureterostomy
Ureteroplasty

DETAILS TO CONSIDER

Patient is older than 70 and/or has comorbidity or complications. The loss of a kidney transplant indicates the need to return to hemodialysis or peritoneal dialysis. Refer to **DRG 303** for care of the patient with a urinary diversion.

POTENTIAL HOME CARE PROBLEMS

1. Health management deficit related to need for long-term medical management. NOTE: loss of transplant receives hemodialysis or peritoneal dialysis. Urinary diversions require long-term care.

2. Alteration in nutrition related to chronic renal failure.

3. Alteration in urine elimination related to diversionary procedures.

4. Self-perception/self-concept related to loss of renal transplant. NOTE: rejection of the transplanted organ may be perceived by the patient as a rejection by the donor. The patient may also view the rejection as a personal failure due to some real or imagined indiscretion. This may lead to profound feelings of guilt, loss of self-esteem and depression.

PLAN

Assess patient's understanding and acceptance of chronic illness. Involve social service for support and financial counseling.

Refer to **DRGs 316** and **317.**

Refer to **DRG 303.**

Offer psychiatric counseling as needed. Encourage patient to verbalize feelings.

REFERRAL INFORMATION

Refer to **DRG 303** for urinary diversion. Refer to **DRG 317** for management of dialysis.

DRG 305

| MDC 11 | RW$ 1.7043 | Surgical | Outlier Cutoff 32 | Mean LOS 11.9 |

Kidney, Ureter and Major Bladder Procedures for Nonmalignancy – Age < 70 w/o CC

OPERATIVE PROCEDURES WITH POTENTIAL HOME CARE NEEDS

Aorticorenal bypass
Nephroureterotomy
Radical cystectomy

Refer to **DRG 304.**

DRG 306

| MDC 11 | RW$ 1.1399 | Surgical | Outlier Cutoff 29 | Mean LOS 8.6 |

Prostatectomy – Age > = 70 and/or CC

OPERATIVE PROCEDURES WITH POTENTIAL HOME CARE NEEDS

Transurethral prostatectomy
Suprapubic prostatectomy
Retropubic prostatectomy
Radical prostatectomy
Perineal prostatectomy

DETAILS TO CONSIDER

Patient is older than 70 and/or has comorbidity and complications. The approach to prostatic surgery is determined based on patient's age and other health limitations, degree of obstruction, cause of lesion and accessibility of the lesion.

POTENTIAL HOME CARE PROBLEMS

1. Health management deficit related to age.
   NOTE: elderly patients are more apt to have other health deficits that impact upon total care needs.

2. Alteration in nutrition related to need for hydration to reduce risk of clotting leading to obstruction and infection.

3. Alteration in elimination related to signs and symptoms affected by surgical procedures.
   NOTE: burning on urination frequently occurs after the indwelling catheter is removed and may last for a period of two weeks.

PLAN

Assess patient's ability to care for self and to carry out activities of daily living.

Instruct patient to drink 2,000–3,000 ml every day depending on cardiac reserve. Instruct patient to avoid consumption of alcohol which causes burning on urination.

To improve urinary control, instruct patient to perform perineal exercises:
- tense the perineal muscles for as long as possible by pressing the buttocks together.
- relax.

Urinary incontinence and dribbling are frequent sequelae to prostatic surgery. They are usually temporary symptoms.

• repeat exercise frequently throughout the day. The patient should also interrupt flow of urine when voiding, hold for a few seconds, then continue to empty bladder. Instruct patient to always void at time of first urge. Instruct patient on methods to protect clothes from soiling while lack of urinary control persists. Many products are available, including external drainage catheters and padded/lined underpants. Instruct patient to keep the skin clean and dry to prevent excoriation and rash.

4. Activity and exercise pattern related to surgery.

Instruct patient to avoid straining and strenuous activity until incision heals to prevent wound separation.

5. Sexuality — related to surgery. NOTE: total prostatectomy may result in impotence due to severence of nerves and muscles involved in penile erection. In some modified procedures this function can be saved.

Offer sexual counseling when indicated. Encourage patient to verbalize feelings and concerns regarding loss of potency.

REFERRAL INFORMATION

Need for referral is based on patient's ability to provide self-care and ability of family to fulfill patient's dependency needs. Referral information should include: teaching plan for regaining bladder control; skin care measures to protect from irritation due to incontinence; method utilized to manage urinary incontinence; hydration measures; equipment and supplies needed to manage incontinence, such as disposable bed pans, external catheters, diapers; and patient's acceptance of illness and prognosis.

DRG 307

MDC 11	RW$ 0.9513	Surgical	Outlier Cutoff 26	Mean LOS 7.2

Prostatectomy – Age < 70 w/o CC

OPERATIVE PROCEDURES WITH POTENTIAL HOME CARE NEEDS

Transurethral prostatectomy
Suprapubic prostatectomy
Retropubic prostatectomy
Radical prostatectomy
Perineal prostatectomy

See **DRG 306.**

POTENTIAL HOME CARE PROBLEM

Sexuality related to surgery. NOTE: partial prostatectomy does not usually result in impotence. Bilateral vasectomy is sometimes performed at time of prostatectomy to reduce risk of epididymitis.

PLAN

Instruct patient to refrain from sexual intercourse for 6–8 weeks following surgery to facilitate healing. Encourage patient to express feelings related to sterility and inability to reproduce. Involve patient's wife. Provide for social service and/or sexual counseling if indicated.

DRG 308

MDC 11	RW$ 1.0441	Surgical	Outlier Cutoff 27	Mean LOS 7.1

Minor Bladder Procedures – Age > = 70 and/or CC

OPERATIVE PROCEDURES WITH POTENTIAL HOME CARE NEEDS

Cystotomy
Bladder biopsy
Cystocele repair
Partial cystectomy

DETAILS TO CONSIDER

Patient is older than 70 and/or has comorbidity or complications.

POTENTIAL HOME CARE PROBLEMS	PLAN
1. Health management deficit related to age and surgical insult.	Assess patient's ability to function at same level of independence as prior to hospitalization.
2. Alteration in urine elimination related to surgery.	Assess patient's ability to maintain urinary continence. If patient does not have urine control, instruct in measures to manage incontinence. Refer to **DRG 306.**
3. Alteration in stool elimination related to surgery. NOTE: following cystocele repair, constipation may result from need to prevent straining to allow for healing of incision line.	Instruct patient in dietary measures to promote normal bowel elimination. Stool softener medications may be prescribed to prevent straining.

REFERRAL INFORMATION

Need for referral depends on patient's ability to resume self-care and family's ability to fulfill dependency needs. Reinstate services which were present prior to hospitalization.

DRG 309

MDC 11	RW$ 0.9290	Surgical	Outlier Cutoff 26	Mean LOS 5.7

Minor Bladder Procedures – Age < 70 w/o CC

Same as **DRG 308.**

Transurethral Procedures – Age > = 70 and/or CC

OPERATIVE PROCEDURES WITH POTENTIAL HOME CARE NEEDS

Transurethral bladder biopsy
Removal of ureter obstruction
Transurethral adhesiolysis

DETAILS TO CONSIDER

Patient is older than 70 and/or with comorbidity or complications. Any manipulation of the urinary tract predisposes the patient to increased risk for urinary tract infection.

POTENTIAL HOME CARE PROBLEM

Alteration in elimination related to surgery. See **DRG 306** for management of incontinence/dribbling.

PLAN

In order to reduce risk of UTI:
- instruct patient to drink 2–3,000 ml of fluids every day depending on cardiac status.
- instruct patient to void at first urge.
- instruct patient to cleanse urethral meatus after each voiding/defecation.
- instruct patient to promptly report signs and symptoms of UTI to physician, i.e. dysuria, burning, frequency, urgency, change in volume, color, odor hematuria, presence of mucous shreds in urine, incontinence and pneumaturia.

REFERRAL INFORMATION

If patient was receiving home care services, reinstate services. New referral depends on development of self-care deficits resulting from surgery. Referral information should include management of incontinence.

See **DRG 306**.

Transurethral Procedures – Age < 70 w/o CC

Same as **DRG 310**.

DRG 312

MDC 11	RW$ 0.7424	Surgical	Outlier Cutoff 22	Mean LOS 5.2

Urethral Procedures – Age > = 70 and/or CC

OPERATIVE PROCEDURES WITH POTENTIAL HOME CARE NEEDS

Urethrotomy
Urethral meatotomy
Urethral reconstruction
Urethral stricture release

DETAILS TO CONSIDER

Patient is older than 70 and/or with comorbidity or complications. See **DRG 306** for management of incontinence/dribbling. See **DRG 310** for prevention of UTI.

POTENTIAL HOME CARE PROBLEMS

1. Health management deficit related to urethral stricture. NOTE: dilatations of urethra may be accomplished via passage of urethral stones of increasing size over a prolonged period of time.

2. Alteration in urine elimination related to stricture of urethra.

PLAN

Assess patient's ability to adhere to prolonged medical management to achieve goal of normal urinary elimination.

Instruct patient to take warm water sitz baths to facilitate initiation of voiding as well as to reduce dysuria and burning sensations which may persist for several weeks following procedures.

REFERRAL INFORMATION

Refer to **DRG 310.**

DRG 313

MDC 11	RW$ 0.6897	Surgical	Outlier Cutoff 21	Mean LOS 5.1

Urethral Procedures – Age 18–69 w/o CC

Same as **DRG 312.**

| MDC 11 | RW$ 0.4368 | Surgical | Outlier Cutoff 11 | Mean LOS 2.3 |

Urethral Procedures – Age 0–17

OPERATIVE PROCEDURES WITH POTENTIAL HOME CARE NEEDS

Same as **DRG 313.**

Hypospadias repair

DETAILS TO CONSIDER

Refer to **DRG 312.** Refer to pediatric texts for specific information.

| MDC 11 | RW$ 2.4884 | Surgical | Outlier Cutoff 30 | Mean LOS 9.8 |

Other Kidney and Urinary Tract Operating Room Procedures

OPERATIVE PROCEDURES WITH POTENTIAL HOME CARE NEEDS

Revise renal dialysis shunt
Insert vessel to vessel cannula

DETAILS TO CONSIDER

Refer to **DRGs 304** and **317.**

POTENTIAL HOME CARE PROBLEMS

1a. Health management deficit related to creation and maintenance of arteriovenous (A-V) fistula or shunt. NOTE: the usual site for the creation of an A-V fistula or shunt is the brachial or cephalic vessels in the forearm. A fistula is an internal A-V connection constructed autologously or with bovine or synthetic materials, whereas a shunt is an external A-V connection made from synthetic materials.

PLAN

Instruct patient to palpate fistula for characteristic bruit to ensure continued patency of fistula or shunt. Instruct patient to avoid constricting clothing and/or jewelry over extremity with fistula or shunt. Instruct patient with shunt on performance of meticulous wound management techniques to prevent site infections. Instruct patients to avoid intravenous infusion venipunctures and blood pressure measurements on the extremity with fistula or shunt. Instruct patient to wear a Medic-Alert bracelet identifying extremity with fistula or shunt. Instruct patient to perform strengthening exercises such as squeezing resistive devices. This will help to improve integrity of vasculature for hemodialysis. Instruct patient with shunt to always carry bulldog clamps to clamp tubing if an accidental disruption in tubing should occur.

1b. Health management deficit related to placement of peritoneal catheters for peritoneal dialysis.

Instruct patient in protocols for care of peritoneal catheters. NOTE: meticulous care of catheters is essential in order to prevent fixed site infections and peritonitis.

2. Self-perception/self-concept deficit related to alteration in body image due to presence of A-V fistula, A-V shunt or peritoneal catheters.

Encourage patient to verbalize feelings regarding presence of A-V fistula or peritoneal catheter and how this affects physical appearance and sexuality. Suggest clothing that will disguise and protect fistula or catheter.

REFERRAL INFORMATION

Need for referral depends on status of renal failure and patient's ability to perform self-care measures. Nursing evaluation and care may be performed at time of dialysis treatment. Inform the home care nurse of protocols for care of A-V shunts, fistula or peritoneal catheters.

DRG 316

MDC 11	RW$ 1.3314	Medical	Outlier Cutoff 27	Mean LOS 6.7

Renal Failure w/o Dialysis

DIAGNOSTIC PROCEDURES WITH POTENTIAL HOME CARE NEEDS

Acute renal failure
Chronic renal failure

DETAILS TO CONSIDER

Acute or chronic renal failure without dialysis requires strict adherence to medical management regimen. All efforts are directed towards optimizing remaining renal function and minimizing workload placed on renal system.

The etiology of the acute or chronic renal failure impacts upon prognosis and progression of disease. Acute renal failure resulting from renal toxins is usually reversible while renal failure induced by vascular disease is not. Chronic renal failure connotes life-long medical management and increased potential for other organ system failures.

POTENTIAL HOME CARE PROBLEMS

1. Health management deficit related to potential major alteration in lifestyle and health status.

PLAN

Assess patient's acceptance of illness and ability to comply with medical management regime. Involve social service for counseling.

2. Alteration in nutrition related to dietary restrictions. NOTE: protein, sodium, potassium and fluid volume restrictions are usual.

Initiate dietary instructions and obtain feedback from patient to assess understanding of diet prescription. Assess impact of patient's restricted diet on other family members and ability of food preparer to adapt menu to meet the patient's dietary regime. Assess patient's state of nutrition and appetite. NOTE: anorexia is associated with uremia.

3. Alteration in elimination related to decreased renal function creating potential for fluid retention.

Teach patient how to calculate intake and output to assess daily fluid balance. Teach patient to measure weight at the same time each day. Teach patient to assess for pedal, sacral and orbital edema.

4. Activity and exercise related to decreased energy level and bone disease. NOTE: rising blood urea nitrogen (BUN) levels create mental status changes and lethargy.

Assess patient's activity tolerance. Assistive ambulation devices may be necessary for mobility. Assess patient's ability to safely perform activities of daily living and self-care measures.

5. Self-perception/self-concept related to loss of independence and need for role changes.

Assess patient for loss of self-esteem due to dependence on others for daily care. Encourage patient to verbalize feelings. Involve social service for counseling with patient and family for major lifestyle adjustments.

6. Sexuality-reproduction related to uremia. NOTE: impotence, decreased libido, menstrual irregularities and sterility are often sequelae of uremia.

Provide opportunity for sexual counseling if indicated.

REFERRAL INFORMATION

Referral information should include:

- background data.
- course of hospitalization.
- predicted prognosis and health status goals.
- medical management regime.
- patient's acceptance of chronic nature of renal failure.
- teaching protocols utilized in patient education.

Durable medical equipment needs are dependent upon patient's health status. Potential needs include walker, cane, wheelchair and hospital bed.

DRG 317

MDC 11	RW$ 0.2385	Medical	Outlier Cutoff 3	Mean LOS 1.2

Renal Failure with Dialysis

DIAGNOSTIC PROCEDURE WITH POTENTIAL HOME CARE NEEDS

Admission for renal dialysis
After care-dialysis

DETAILS TO CONSIDER

Hospitalization admission under this DRG most often connotes cardiac vascular instability during or after dialysis requiring observation and nursing/medical management. Fluid volume shifts and electrolyte imbalances generally are the common areas of concern.

Refer to **DRGs 315** and **316.**

POTENTIAL HOME CARE PROBLEMS

1. Health management deficit related to need for dialysis treatments on a routine basis, most often scheduled 2–3 times each week.

2. Ability to cope/stress tolerance related to dialysis routines. NOTE: many patients have difficulty adjusting to their dependency on dialysis for life-support, requiring 4–6 hours treatment 2–3 times every week.

3. Activity and exercise deficit related to hemodialysis regimen. NOTE: patient may experience cyclic changes in physical well-being related to hemodialysis schedule. In postdialysis the patient may feel weak, followed by an increasing sense of well-being over the next 24–48 hours. This period is followed by a deterioration in strength, appetite and sense of well-being related to the accumulation of body wastes, signifying the need for another dialysis treatment. The cycle repeats itself. Continuous peritoneal dialysis may avert these symptoms.

4. Alteration in nutrition related to dialysis management. NOTE: dietary restrictions for hemodialysis patients are more stringent than for the peritoneal dialysis patient because there is greater loss of protein and fluid through the peritoneal membrane. Peritoneal dialysis allows for more freedom in food selections.

PLAN

Ascertain and assist with transportation arrangements to the dialysis center in order to meet scheduled appointments. Involve social service to assist with financial arrangements. NOTE: all dialysis patients may apply for Medicare reimbursement.

Involve social service for counseling. Encourage patient to verbalize feelings.

Instruct patient that cyclic changes may be minimized by strict adherence to the medical/nursing regimen, with particular adherence to diet and fluid restriction.

Involve the dietitian in discharge diet instructions. Obtain feedback from patient and family regarding their understanding and appreciation of the importance of dietary management.

REFERRAL INFORMATION

Nursing evaluation and monitoring may be accomplished during routine dialysis treatments. If more frequent observation or other self-care needs exist, a home care nurse referral may be indicated. If patient is to be maintained on home dialysis, coordinate needs for home care with participating dialysis unit and social service. Durable medical equipment needs may include: hospital bed or recliner may be necessary to facilitate home dialysis regimen; blood pressure device and stethoscope for blood pressure monitoring for the home dialysis patient; and assistive ambulatory devices.

MDC 11   **RW$ 0.9142**   **Medical**   **Outlier Cutoff 26**   **Mean LOS 5.5**

Kidney and Urinary Tract Neoplasms – Age > = 70 and/or CC

DIAGNOSTIC PROCEDURES WITH POTENTIAL HOME CARE NEEDS

Malignancy of any structure in system
Kidney
Ureter
Bladder
Urethra

DETAILS TO CONSIDER

Patient is older than 70 with comorbidity or complications.

Refer to **DRG 303.**

POTENTIAL HOME CARE PROBLEM

Activity and exercise deficit related to renal
biopsy procedure.

PLAN

Instruct patient to avoid strenuous activity or
heavy lifting for a minimum of two weeks after
biopsy.

REFERRAL INFORMATION

Due to malignancy and age over 70 a home care referral is indicated. Hospice home care or oncology
programs may be instituted.

MDC 11   **RW$ 0.7942**   **Medical**   **Outlier Cutoff 24**   **Mean LOS 4.2**

Kidney and Urinary Tract Neoplasms – Age < 70 w/o CC

Same as **DRG 318.**

DRG 320

Kidney and Urinary Tract Infections – Age > = 70 and/or CC

DIAGNOSTIC PROCEDURES WITH POTENTIAL HOME CARE NEEDS

TB of organs
Syphilis of kidney
Chronic pyelonephritis
Renal abscess
Acute cystitis

DETAILS TO CONSIDER

Patient is older than 70 and/or with comorbidity or complications. Patient is at risk for infection to recur, particularly if underlying cause is not adequately treated. Many urinary tract infections (UTI) are asymptomatic.

POTENTIAL HOME CARE PROBLEMS

PLAN

1. Health management deficit related to need for long-term medical follow-up.

Encourage patient to provide follow-up urine specimens for screening and culture, even though they may be asymptomatic. Encourage adherence to medication schedules. NOTE: medication routines may be long-term, such as 2 or more years for the treatment of TB. Involve social service for financial concerns.

2. Alteration in urine elimination related to prevention of recurrent UTI.

Instruct patient to drink 2–3,000 ml of fluid every day depending on cardiac status. Instruct patient to void at first urge and at least every 3 hours during the day.

3. Alteration in sexuality related to UTI associated with sexual intercourse.

Instruct female patients to empty bladder immediately after sexual intercourse to clear meatus.

4. Knowledge deficit related to hygiene measures.

Instruct female patients to cleanse urinary meatus and perineal area after each bowel movement by cleansing from front to back. Avoid tub baths. Showers are preferred in patients at risk for repeated UTIs.

REFERRAL INFORMATION

Reinstate prior services. A referral may be indicated for monitoring compliance with medication and hygiene measures.

MDC 11	RW$ 0.6803	Medical	Outlier Cutoff 23	Mean LOS 5.6

Kidney and Urinary Tract Infections – Age 18–69 w/o CC

Same as **DRG 320.**

DRG 322

MDC 11	RW$ 0.4553	Medical	Outlier Cutoff 13	Mean LOS 3.7

Kidney and Urinary Tract Infections – Age 0–17

Same as **DRG 320.**

DETAILS TO CONSIDER

Refer to **DRG 320.** Refer to pediatric texts for specific information.

DRG 323

MDC 11	RW$ 0.7131	Medical	Outlier Cutoff 25	Mean LOS 4.9

Urinary Stones – Age > = 70 and/or CC

DIAGNOSTIC PROCEDURES WITH POTENTIAL HOME CARE NEEDS

Calculus of kidney, ureter or bladder
Hydronephrosis
Ureteric obstruction

DETAILS TO CONSIDER

Patient is over 70 with comorbidity and complications. Obstruction in the urinary tract predisposes to infection. Refer to **DRG 320.** Frequent or chronic obstruction to urine flow may cause permanent kidney damage.

POTENTIAL HOME CARE PROBLEMS

1. Alteration in nutrition related to dietary management to prevent or retard stone formation. NOTE: most renal calculi are compounds containing calcium, magnesium, phosphates and oxalates.

PLAN

Instruct patient in a moderately reduced calcium and phosphorus diet. Advise patient to reduce intake of milk and vitamin D. Vitamin A may be supplemented in diet.

2. Alteration in elimination related to stone formation. NOTE: concentrated urine predisposes to urolithiasis.

Encourage patient to drink 2–3,000 ml of fluids every day. Teach patient to monitor intake/output balance.

3. Activity and exercise pattern related to stone formation.

Encourage patient to exercise and to avoid long periods of inactivity.

4. Pain tolerance related to urolithiasis.

Instruct patient to strain urine for calculi upon initiation of characteristic colicky pain. Pain may radiate to testes in males and to perineum in females.

REFERRAL INFORMATION

Reinstate prior services. Referral may be indicated to monitor compliance with dietary regimen and to reinforce health teaching in preventive measures.

DRG 324

MDC 11	RW$ 0.5472	Medical	Outlier Cutoff 19	Mean LOS 3.9

Urinary Stones – Age < 70 w/o CC

Same as **DRG 323.**

DRG 325

MDC 11	RW$ 0.7247	Medical	Outlier Cutoff 25	Mean LOS 5.4

Kidney and Urinary Tract Signs and Symptoms Age > = 70 and/or CC

DIAGNOSTIC PROCEDURES WITH POTENTIAL HOME CARE NEEDS

Hematuria
Dysuria
Urethral discharge

DETAILS TO CONSIDER

Patient is over 70 and/or with comorbidity and complications.

Refer to **DRG 320.**

| MDC 11 | RW$ 0.5875 | Medical | Outlier Cutoff 21 | Mean LOS 4.3 |

Kidney and Urinary Tract Signs and Symptoms Age 18–69 w/o CC

Same as **DRG 326.**

Refer to **DRG 320.**

| MDC 11 | RW$ 0.5027 | Medical | Outlier Cutoff 14 | Mean LOS 3.1 |

Kidney and Urinary Tract Signs and Symptoms – Age 0–17

Same as **DRG 325.**

DETAILS TO CONSIDER

Refer to **DRG 320.** Refer to pediatric texts for specific information. Congenital malformations may predispose to signs and symptoms.

| MDC 11 | RW$ 0.6508 | Medical | Outlier Cutoff 22 | Mean LOS 4.8 |

Urethral Stricture – Age > = 70 and /or CC

DIAGNOSTIC PROCEDURE WITH POTENTIAL HOME CARE NEEDS

Urethral stricture

DETAILS TO CONSIDER

Patient is over 70 and/or with comorbidity or complications. Refer to **DRG 312.** Obstructions to urinary flow predisposes to urinary tract infections. Refer to **DRG 320.**

DRG 329

| MDC 11 | RW$ 0.5326 | Medical | Outlier Cutoff 17 | Mean LOS 3.9 |

Urethral Stricture – Age 18–69 w/o CC

Refer to **DRGs** 312 and 320.

DRG 330

| MDC 11 | RW$ 0.2817 | Medical | Outlier Cutoff 5 | Mean LOS 1.6 |

Urethral Stricture – Age 0–17

DIAGNOSTIC PROCEDURE WITH POTENTIAL HOME CARE NEEDS

Urethral stricture

DETAILS TO CONSIDER

Refer to **DRGs** 312 and 320. Refer to pediatric texts for specific information.

DRG 331

| MDC 11 | RW$ 0.8919 | Medical | Outlier Cutoff 26 | Mean LOS 6.3 |

Other Kidney and Urinary Tract Diagnoses – Age $>= 70$ and/or CC

DIAGNOSTIC PROCEDURES WITH POTENTIAL HOME CARE NEEDS

Kidney injury
Impaired renal function
Irradiation cystitis

DETAILS TO CONSIDER

Patient is over 70 and/or with comorbidity and complications. Trauma to kidneys may produce temporary or chronic renal failure. Refer to **DRGs** 316, 317, and 320.

MDC 11	RW$ 0.7763	Medical	Outlier Cutoff 25	Mean LOS 5.0

Other Kidney and Urinary Tract Diagnoses – Age 18–69 w/o CC

Same as **DRG 331.**

MDC 11	RW$ 0.5146	Medical	Outlier Cutoff 18	Mean LOS 3.2

Other Kidney and Urinary Tract Diagnoses – Age 0–17

DIAGNOSTIC PROCEDURES WITH POTENTIAL HOME CARE NEEDS

Same as **DRG 331.**

Congenital anomaly of kidney and urinary tract

DETAILS TO CONSIDER

Refer to **DRG 331.** Refer to pediatric texts for specific information.

12 MDC 12 DISEASES AND DISORDERS OF THE MALE REPRODUCTIVE SYSTEM

SURGICAL GROUPINGS (12 DRGs)

Major Pelvic Procedures

Transurethral Prostatectomy

Testes Procedures

Penis Procedures

Circumcision

Other OR Procedures

MEDICAL GROUPINGS (7 DRGs)

Malignancy

Benign Prostatic Hypertrophy

Inflammation

Sterilization

Other Diagnoses

MASTER HOME CARE PLANNING GUIDE
FOR DISEASES AND DISORDERS OF THE
MALE REPRODUCTIVE SYSTEM

Pattern	Assessment Factors	Plan
1. Health management deficit	Assess patient's ability to care for self and effect of illness on job status. In some diagnoses the care of an ostomy, tube or catheter may be required.	Assess patient's ability to carry out procedures required. If a procedure such as ostomy care or catheter care is required, give patient detailed written instructions. Include caregiver in teaching.
2. Alteration in elimination	Assess effect of diagnosis and procedure on ability to void normally. Assess long-term effect of change in urination such as urinary diversion procedures, suprapubic tubes or intermittent catheterization.	See specific DRG.
3. Cognitive/perceptual pattern: 3a. alteration in comfort	Assess amount of pain and plan for control, especially in malignancies and inflammatory diseases.	Instruct patient in pain relieving measures. See specific DRG.
3b. knowledge deficit related to disease process	Determine expected problems associated with the disease process, such as blood in urine, decreasing stream or testicular spasm.	Teach patient what to expect and what symptoms require mechanical attention on an emergency basis. See specific DRG.
4. Body image disturbance	Assess outcome of diagnosis or procedure and discuss change patient perceives in body image. Determine if there will be a negative effect on the patient or a positive effect.	If there will be a negative effect, refer both patient and significant other to counseling.
5. Role-relationship alteration	As in Pattern #4, assess possibility of a negative effect such as loss of sexual function or loss of ability to carry out normal job.	See specific DRG.

MDC 12   **RW$ 1.5612**   **Surgical**   **Outlier Cutoff 30**   **Mean LOS 12.7**

Major Male Pelvic Procedures with CC

OPERATIVE PROCEDURE WITH POTENTIAL HOME CARE NEEDS

Total cystectomy

DETAILS TO CONSIDER

Total cystectomy requires a urinary diversion and may include resection of local pelvic nodes, prostate, seminal vesicles and urethra. The surgery may be performed in two operations with urinary diversion and staging first and cystectomy later, or as one total procedure. It may also be done following radiation therapy. The procedure may be done for a malignancy or for a neurogenic bladder.

POTENTIAL HOME CARE PROBLEMS

PLAN

1. Health management deficit.

Depending on type of diversion, the patient will need detailed instructions in self-care. If the patient had a neurogenic bladder because of spinal cord disease, the self-care of the urinary diversion will be one part of the patient's overall self-care routine. Setting up an easy to follow routine is especially important for patients with other health problems.

2. Alteration in elimination.

Patient may have one of these types of urinary diversions:
- ileal loop (ureteroileal-cutaneous)
- colon loop (ureterocolic-cutaneous)
- rectal bladder (ureterorectal with colostomy fecal diversion)
- uretero-cutaneous

Detailed instructions will be needed by the patient and caregiver with self-teaching prior to discharge. If the patient has an ostomy, establish a pattern for ostomy appliance management, skin care, set-up for night drainage and odor control.

3. Role-relationship pattern changes.

The patient and significant other will need counseling if it is determined that sexual activity will be affected.

REFERRAL INFORMATION

Referral for home care nurse for management of urinary diversion and monitoring progression of disease is indicated. Equipment needs for the ostomate should be detailed and equipment ordered and delivered before discharge. Referral to an enterostomal therapist is necessary for long-term management in some cases.

DRG 335

MDC 12   RW$ 1.3590   Surgical   Outlier Cutoff 29   Mean LOS 11.8

Major Male Pelvic Procedures w/o CC

See **DRG 334.**

DRG 336

MDC 12   RW$ 1.0079   Surgical   Outlier Cutoff 22   Mean LOS 8.4

Transurethral Prostatectomy – Age > = 70 and/or CC

OPERATIVE PROCEDURE WITH POTENTIAL HOME CARE NEEDS
Transurethral prostatectomy

DETAILS TO CONSIDER
This relatively frequent procedure is usually done for a benign condition. At the time of discharge, the patient will be voiding normally, and unless the patient has a complication or comorbidity that renders him unstable, a referral will not be needed.

POTENTIAL HOME CARE PROBLEMS

1. Health management deficit.

2. Alteration in elimination secondary to operative procedure.

PLAN

Instruct patient in signs and symptoms of potential complications, especially the potential of post-op bleeding several days after the procedure. Do not alarm the patient, but discuss the importance of contacting his physician if he experiences bladder pain, spasm, change in color of urine or blood in urine. See **DRG 344.**

Some patients may experience postprostatectomy incontinence. Encourage the patient to discuss this problem, if it occurs, with the physician. If necessary, assist patient in selection of supplies to care for incontinence such as incontinence pants and external catheter. The physician may use other methods if the incontinence problem continues for more than six months. Options include surgical intervention, electrical stimulation devices, medication and perineal exercise.

| MDC 12 | RW$ 0.8491 | Surgical | Outlier Cutoff 17 | Mean LOS 7.2 |

Transurethral Prostatectomy – Age < 70 w/o CC

See **DRG 336.**

| MDC 12 | RW$ 0.9069 | Surgical | Outlier Cutoff 26 | Mean LOS 6.3 |

Testes Procedures, for Malignancy

OPERATIVE PROCEDURES WITH POTENTIAL HOME CARE NEEDS

Testes diagnostic procedure
Unilateral and bilateral orchidectomy
Epididymectomy

DETAILS TO CONSIDER

Patient's long-term needs will depend on prognosis.

POTENTIAL HOME CARE PROBLEM

Alteration in self-concept and alteration in role-relationship pattern.

PLAN

Refer for counseling, especially for patients of childbearing age if diagnosis and procedure will render patient sterile.

REFERRAL INFORMATION

Patients in this group may not have home care needs at the time of discharge, but a referral for follow-up care secondary to the diagnosis of a malignancy should be made.

DRG 339

MDC 12   **RW$ 0.6093**   **Surgical**   **Outlier Cutoff 15**   **Mean LOS 4.5**

Testes Procedures, Nonmalignant – Age > = 18

OPERATIVE PROCEDURES WITH POTENTIAL HOME CARE NEEDS

Excision of hydrocele
Orchiopexy
Cord, epididymis and vas deferens procedures

DETAILS TO CONSIDER

These procedures are usually done as elective procedures; thus home care needs are planned prior to admission.

DRG 340

MDC 12   **RW$ 0.4381**   **Surgical**   **Outlier Cutoff 7**   **Mean LOS 2.4**

Testes Procedures, Nonmalignant – Age 0–17

See **DRG 339**.

DETAILS TO CONSIDER

Evaluation of the family situation and ability to care for the child should be done; if necessary, the parents or guardian should be given assistance in setting up care if both parents will be unavailable for periods of time. The reader is referred to pediatric texts for further information.

MDC 12	RW$ 0.9983	Surgical	Outlier Cutoff 23	Mean LOS 6.0

Penis Procedures

OPERATIVE PROCEDURES WITH POTENTIAL HOME CARE NEEDS

Hypospadias repair
Urethral reconstruction
Penile repair
Insertion of penile prosthesis

DETAILS TO CONSIDER

Some of these procedures are done as elective cases and adequate follow-up can be done by the physician.

POTENTIAL HOME CARE PROBLEM	PLAN
Alteration in self-concept secondary to penile injury.	If trauma is the source of the problem, the patient will need counseling.

REFERRAL INFORMATION

See **DRG 336** for discussion of postoperative incontinence.

MDC 12	RW$ 0.4228	Surgical	Outlier Cutoff 10	Mean LOS 2.8

Circumcision – Age > = 18

OPERATIVE PROCEDURE WITH POTENTIAL HOME CARE NEEDS

Circumcision

DETAILS TO CONSIDER

This is an elective procedure, and follow-up is usually managed in the physician's office.

MDC 12	RW$ 0.3828	Surgical	Outlier Cutoff 4	Mean LOS 1.7

Circumcision – Age 0–17

See **DRG 342.**

DRG 344

MDC 12	RW$ 1.1204	Surgical	Outlier Cutoff 27	Mean LOS 7.4

Other Male Reproductive System Operating Room Procedures for Malignancy

OPERATIVE PROCEDURES WITH POTENTIAL HOME CARE NEEDS

Formation of cystostomy
Closure of cystostomy
Bladder lesion destruction
Control postoperative prostatectomy hemorrhage

See **DRGs 334** and **336.**

DETAILS TO CONSIDER

In patients with formation of a cystostomy, extensive education on self-care will be needed. Those with closure will not need instruction in self-care.

POTENTIAL HOME CARE PROBLEM

Health management deficit.

PLAN

If there is a new cystostomy, instruct the patient in self-care. See **DRG 334.** Needs will depend on procedure and method of urinary drainage.

REFERRAL INFORMATION

Patients in this group have a malignancy as an underlying diagnosis; therefore a referral for follow-up is indicated.

DRG 345

MDC 12	RW$ 0.8334	Surgical	Outlier Cutoff 26	Mean LOS 5.6

Other Male Reproductive System Operating Room Procedures Except for Malignancy

OPERATIVE PROCEDURES WITH POTENTIAL HOME CARE NEEDS

Biopsy of reproduction structures

DETAILS TO CONSIDER

Long-term needs will depend on outcome of biopsy and location of lesion and reason for biopsy since this DRG does not cover malignancy.

| MDC 12 | RW$ 0.9395 | Medical | Outlier Cutoff 27 | Mean LOS 6.9 |

Malignancy, Male Reproductive System – Age > = 70 and/or CC

PRINCIPAL DIAGNOSIS WITH POTENTIAL HOME CARE NEEDS

Malignancy, male reproductive system

DETAILS TO CONSIDER

Long-term needs in this group will depend on stage of disease, location of malignancy and method of treatment.

| MDC 12 | RW$ 0.8304 | Medical | Outlier Cutoff 26 | Mean LOS 5.7 |

Malignancy, Male Reproductive System – Age < 70 w/o CC

See **DRG 346.**

| MDC 12 | RW$ 0.8864 | Medical | Outlier Cutoff 26 | Mean LOS 6.2 |

Benign Prostatic Hypertrophy – Age > = 70 and/or CC

PRINCIPAL DIAGNOSIS WITH POTENTIAL HOME CARE NEEDS

Benign prostatic hypertrophy

DETAILS TO CONSIDER

Since this is a medical group the follow-up needs will depend on nonsurgical measures.

POTENTIAL HOME CARE PROBLEMS

1. Health management deficit.

PLAN

Instruct patient in conservative measures for controlling prostatic congestion such as frequent intercourse. The physician may include prostatic massage on a regular basis in the plan of care.

2. Alteration in elimination.

Instruct patient in fluid management to prevent pressure on ureters and kidneys such as avoidance of excessive fluid intake in a short period of time and urination when the urge is first felt. Instruct the patient about the diuretic effect of alcohol which, when combined with increased fluid intake, may lead to urinary retention that may need medical intervention.

REFERRAL INFORMATION

Follow-up care can usually be managed in the physician's office.

DRG 349

MDC 12	RW$ 0.6998	Medical	Outlier Cutoff 22	Mean LOS 4.9

Benign Prostatic Hypertrophy – Age < 70 w/o CC

See **DRG 348.**

DRG 350

MDC 12	RW$ 0.6096	Medical	Outlier Cutoff 20	Mean LOS 5.2

Inflammation of the Male Reproductive System

PRINCIPAL DIAGNOSES WITH POTENTIAL HOME CARE NEEDS

TB of structures
Genital herpes
Orchitis
Gonorrhea
Urogenital trichomonas
Venereal disease
Prostatitis

DETAILS TO CONSIDER

The long-term needs of patients in this group depend on the clinical manifestations of the disease. For more information see DRG that includes the clinical manifestations exhibited by the patient.

REFERRAL INFORMATION

Some of the diagnoses in this group are reportable since they are communicable. Follow-up case finding in contacts is necessary. Consult the health department in your area to determine methods of case reporting and discuss the reporting and case finding with the physician.

MDC 12	RW$ 0.2655	Medical	Outlier Cutoff 3	Mean LOS 1.3

Sterilization, Male

DETAILS TO CONSIDER

A medical admission for sterilization is very rare!

MDC 12	RW$ 0.6385	Medical	Outlier Cutoff 20	Mean LOS 4.4

Other Male Reproductive System Diagnoses

PRINCIPAL DIAGNOSES WITH POTENTIAL HOME CARE NEEDS

Benign neoplasm of testes
Male infertility
Injury to external genitalia
Undescended testicle
Priapism

See **DRG 341.**

DETAILS TO CONSIDER

Long-term needs depend on outcome of medical therapy and/or effect of condition on ability to urinate or establish fertility. In admissions for priapism the cause of the problem needs to be investigated and long-term follow-up initiated depending on the cause. For example, sickle-cell anemia may be the underlying cause which needs long-term follow-up.

13 MDC 13
DISEASES AND DISORDERS OF THE FEMALE REPRODUCTIVE SYSTEM

SURGICAL GROUPINGS (13 DRGs)

Pelvic Evisceration and Vulvectomy

Radical and Nonradical Hysterectomy

Reconstructive Procedures

Uterus and Adnexa Procedures

Tubal Interruption

Vagina, Cervix and Vulva Procedures

Laparoscopy and Endoscopy

Laparoscopic Tubal Interruption

D and C Conization

Other OR Procedures

MEDICAL GROUPINGS (4 DRGs)

Malignancy

Infections

Menstrual and Other Disorders

MASTER HOME CARE PLANNING GUIDE FOR DISEASES AND DISORDERS OF THE FEMALE REPRODUCTIVE SYSTEM

Pattern	Assessment Factors	Plan
1. Health management deficit	Length of time of health care (posthospital) depends on procedure and prognosis. Because pelvic muscles are used in lifting objects and activities such as stair climbing, assessment of home environment, home and work responsibilities is indicated. Many of these procedures are done as elective procedures; thus the patient will have made arrangements for care prior to admission.	See specific DRG.
2. Alteration in elimination	Bowel and bladder functions may be involved because of close proximity of these organs to the female reproductive organs.	See specific DRG.
3. Alteration in hormone balance	If ovaries are removed, determine plan for replacement therapy from physician.	Instruct patient to follow-up with physician for replacement therapy. Since not all physicians manage the replacement of female hormones the same, individual follow-up is essential. All patients should be informed of the need for calcium and vitamin D supplements to prevent osteoporosis. Instruct patient in normal body changes to be expected following oophorectomy. Instruct patient in breast self-examination.
4. Alteration in self-concept, body image, sexuality and reproductive function	The effect of diagnosis of any type on the female reproductive system has implications for the woman. The seriousness of the condition and the effect on reproduction or sexual function and the method of treatment has an impact on the woman no matter what age.	Counseling may be needed. See specific DRG.

REFERRAL INFORMATION

Many of these procedures are done on an elective basis; therefore the patient and caregiver should have prior arrangements for follow-up home care. If the patient is caregiver to another person or persons, assistance may be needed. Information on continued need for follow-up screening should be given.

Pelvic Evisceration, Radical Hysterectomy and Vulvectomy

OPERATIVE PROCEDURES WITH POTENTIAL HOME CARE NEEDS

Pelvic evisceration
Radical hysterectomy
Vulvectomy

DETAILS TO CONSIDER

In pelvic evisceration, all of the organs in the pelvic area are involved including the bladder and bowel. In a radical hysterectomy, all of the female reproductive organs are involved including the uterus, Fallopian tubes, ovaries and surrounding lymph glands. In vulvectomy, the external female organs are involved but not necessarily the internal organs such as uterus and ovaries.

POTENTIAL HOME CARE PROBLEMS

PLAN

1. Alteration in elimination.

If the patient has a colostomy refer to **DRG 146** and **DRG 147**. If the patient has a urinary diversion refer to **DRG 303**.

2. Self-care deficit.

Assess patient's ability to plan and organize own care. Include primary caregiver in procedures. Have enterostomal therapist work with patient to determine appropriate equipment. This is especially important if patient has more than one type of ostomy to deal with.

3. Alteration in hormonal balance.

Determine physician plan for postsurgery hormonal therapy. Counsel patient and caregiver on expected changes as a result of loss of ovarian hormones.

4. Alteration in role-relationship.

Determine patient's need for sexual counseling. Determine long-term plans regarding creation of vaginal orifice.

REFERRAL INFORMATION

Follow-up referral is indicated if there is an ostomy, even if the patient appears to be competent in self-care. Communicate the patient's present level of self-care, plans for hormone therapy and future surgery. Relate status of ostomy, type of appliance being used, status of perineal wound and method of wound care. Refer to American Cancer Society, if indicated, for support group for patient and family.

IMPORTANT: The need for family counseling must be assessed, especially in situations in which the patient is in the childbearing age group. If the patient's mother took the drug "Diethylstilbestrol (DES)" during pregnancy, and it can be linked to the patient's present condition, the patient and family must be offered counseling.

DRG 354

| MDC 13 | RW$ 1.1108 | Surgical | Outlier Cutoff 20 | Mean LOS 9.6 |

Nonradical Hysterectomy – Age > = 70 and/or CC

OPERATIVE PROCEDURES WITH POTENTIAL HOME CARE NEEDS

Abdominal hysterectomy, subtotal and total
Vaginal hysterectomy

DETAILS TO CONSIDER

The patient's postoperative hormonal therapy will depend on involvement of ovaries, age and medical plan.

POTENTIAL HOME CARE PROBLEMS

1. Alteration in self-care.

2. Alteration in sexuality.

PLAN

The patient should be able to gradually increase activity and be able to resume normal activity in 6–8 weeks. Physician's orders about bathing and lifting should be reinforced. If the patient is caregiver to others, additional help may be needed for moderate to strenuous activity.

Depending on patient's age and lifestyle, patient should be counseled in expected changes. Diagnoses in this group do *not* usually affect patient's sexual activity. There is usually some restriction on intercourse until healing has occurred.

REFERRAL INFORMATION

Patients can normally do self-care. If there is an activity restriction, arrangement for meals may be necessary, such as Meals-on-Wheels. If patient is caregiver to others, assistance in meeting others' needs is required, especially if there is physical activity involved.

DRG 355

| MDC 13 | RW$ 1.0156 | Surgical | Outlier Cutoff 17 | Mean LOS 8.8 |

Nonradical Hysterectomy – Age < 70 w/o CC

OPERATIVE PROCEDURES WITH POTENTIAL HOME CARE NEEDS

Abdominal hysterectomy, subtotal and total
Vaginal hysterectomy

See **DRG 354.**

MDC 13   **RW$ 0.8460**   **Surgical**   **Outlier Cutoff 18**   **Mean LOS 8.1**

Female Reproductive System Reconstructive Procedures

OPERATIVE PROCEDURES WITH POTENTIAL HOME CARE NEEDS

Uterine suspension
Uterus/adnexa repair
Rectocele repair
Cystocele repair

DETAILS TO CONSIDER

Refer to **DRG 354.**

POTENTIAL HOME CARE PROBLEM

Alteration in elimination secondary to surgical procedure.

PLAN

Instruct patient in changes in diet needed to prevent constipation in order to eliminate straining at stool.

MDC 13   **RW$ 1.9188**   **Surgical**   **Outlier Cutoff 34**   **Mean LOS 13.9**

Uterus and Adnexa Procedures for Malignancy

PRINCIPAL DIAGNOSIS WITH POTENTIAL HOME CARE NEEDS

Malignancy of uterus, adnexa, labia, clitoris

SURGICAL PROCEDURES FOR PRINCIPAL DIAGNOSIS

Oophorectomy
Biopsy procedures

See **DRG 353** and **DRG 354.**

DRG 358

| MDC 13 | RW$ 1.0890 | Surgical | Outlier Cutoff 28 | Mean LOS 8.0 |

Uterus and Adnexa Procedures for Nonmalignancy Except Tubal Interruption

REPRESENTATIVE DIAGNOSES

Removal of tube for ectopic pregnancy
Hysterectomy
Fallopian tube diagnostic procedures

See **DRG 354.**

DRG 359

| MDC 13 | RW$ 0.4279 | Surgical | Outlier Cutoff 7 | Mean LOS 2.3 |

Tubal Interruption for Nonmalignancy

REPRESENTATIVE PROCEDURES

Bilateral tubal crushing
Bilateral tubal division

DETAILS TO CONSIDER

These procedures are done for sterilization on an elective basis.

DRG 360

| MDC 13 | RW$ 0.5985 | Surgical | Outlier Cutoff 19 | Mean LOS 4.2 |

Vagina, Cervix and Vulva Procedures

REPRESENTATIVE PROCEDURES

Cervical repair
Repair of fistulae

See **DRG 354** and **DRG 356.**

| MDC 13 | RW$ 0.4864 | Surgical | Outlier Cutoff 10 | Mean LOS 2.6 |

Laparoscopy and Endoscopy (Female) Except Tubal Interruption

REPRESENTATIVE PROCEDURES

Laparoscopy and endoscopy except tubal interruption

DETAILS TO CONSIDER

These procedures are usually done as an elective diagnostic procedure.

| MDC 13 | RW$ 0.3126 | Surgical | Outlier Cutoff 3 | Mean LOS 1.4 |

Laparoscopic Tubal Interruption

REPRESENTATIVE PROCEDURE

Laparoscopic tubal interruption

DETAILS TO CONSIDER

This is a sterilization procedure done on an elective basis. It is sometimes done as a one-day surgical procedure.

DRG 363

MDC 13   **RW$ 0.6516**   **Surgical**   **Outlier Cutoff 18**   **Mean LOS 4.3**

D and C, Conization and Radioimplant for Malignancy

OPERATIVE PROCEDURES WITH POTENTIAL HOME CARE NEEDS

D and C, conization and radioimplant for malignancy

DETAILS TO CONSIDER

These procedures can sometimes be done as one-day surgery. Sexual intercourse should be avoided until advised by the physician.

POTENTIAL HOME CARE PROBLEM	PLAN
Alteration in sexuality.	Assess impact of surgical procedure and diagnosis on the patient and partner. Advise counseling for the childbearing age patient if there will be long-term effect on reproduction.

REFERRAL INFORMATION

The patient should be able to resume normal activity within a short period of time. If the patient has a diagnosis of a malignancy, refer to American Cancer Society for support and additional information.

DRG 364

MDC 13   **RW$ 0.4028**   **Surgical**   **Outlier Cutoff 9**   **Mean LOS 2.6**

D and C, Conization Except for Malignancy

See **DRG 363.**

| MDC 13 | RW$ 1.7965 | Surgical | Outlier Cutoff 33 | Mean LOS 12.7 |

Other Female Reproductive System Operating Room Procedures

OPERATIVE PROCEDURES WITH POTENTIAL HOME CARE NEEDS

Exploratory laparotomy
Revision of cutaneous ureterostomy
Cystostomy closure

DETAILS TO CONSIDER

These are major procedures, and the follow-up will depend on the outcome of the procedure. In an exploratory laparotomy the findings will have a direct effect on long-term needs. For example, if an inoperative cancer was found, the patient will have long-term needs. In the other procedures the patient may have fewer needs at the time of discharge.

| MDC 13 | RW$ 0.8444 | Medical | Outlier Cutoff 25 | Mean LOS 5.2 |

Malignancy, Female Reproductive System – Age > = 70 and or CC

DIAGNOSIS WITH POTENTIAL HOME CARE NEEDS

Malignancy, female reproductive system

DETAILS TO CONSIDER

The patient is over 70 or has a complication or comorbidity. Since there are no surgical procedures or radioimplants in this DRG, the patient's long-term needs will, in most cases, depend on the comorbidity or complication. If this is a new diagnosis for the patient there may be a need for counseling and referral to the American Cancer Society.

| MDC 13 | RW$ 0.5786 | Medical | Outlier Cutoff 24 | Mean LOS 3.5 |

Malignancy, Female Reproductive System – Age < 70 w/o CC

See **DRG 366.**

DRG 368

| MDC 13 | RW$ 0.7944 | Medical | Outlier Cutoff 27 | Mean LOS 6.7 |

Infections, Female Reproductive System

DIAGNOSES WITH POTENTIAL HOME CARE NEEDS

Venereal disease
Genital herpes
TB of reproductive organs
Candidal vulvovaginitis
Bartholin gland abscess

DETAILS TO CONSIDER

Most patients in this group will not have home care needs but will have need for counseling and follow-up care for the infectious disease. Frequently the infectious disease is treated on an outpatient basis unless there is a complication. The nonvenereal diseases can also be treated on an outpatient basis following diagnosis and initiation of antimicrobial therapy.

DRG 369

| MDC 13 | RW$ 0.6959 | Medical | Outlier Cutoff 25 | Mean LOS 5.1 |

Menstrual and Other Female Reproductive System Disorders

DIAGNOSES WITH POTENTIAL HOME CARE NEEDS

Tuboplasty
Ovarian dysfunction
Endometriosis
Uterine prolapse
Dysplasia of cervix
Menopausal disorder
Infertility
Pelvic organ injury
Malfunction of IUD

DETAILS TO CONSIDER

Follow-up needs for the patient with pelvic organ injury will depend on the type of organ injury and the cause of the injury. If the injury resulted from rape, counseling is essential.

14

MDC 14
PREGNANCY, CHILDBIRTH AND THE PUERPERIUM

SURGICAL GROUPINGS (5 DRGs)

Cesarean Section

Vaginal Delivery w/Sterilization and/or D & C

Vaginal Delivery with OR Procedures

Postpartum Diagnosis with OR Procedures

MEDICAL GROUPINGS (10 DRGs)

Vaginal Delivery

Ectopic Pregnancy

Threatened Abortion

Abortion

False Labor

Other Antepartum Diagnoses

Diagnoses in this MDC are usually treated on specialty units in hospitals, such as labor and delivery and postpartum units. The follow-up care usually falls under maternal and child health programs in community agencies. Some diagnoses in this MDC will need follow-up care separate from traditional maternal-child health, but those diagnoses are covered under other DRGs.

The information and description in this MDC is included for completeness of the DRG listing. The reader is referred to maternal-child health reference works for additional information on planning for long-term needs.

DRG 370

MDC 14	RW$ 0.9912	Surgical	Outlier Cutoff 15	Mean LOS 7.6

Cesarean Section with CC

DRG 371

MDC 14	RW$ 0.7535	Surgical	Outlier Cutoff 10	Mean LOS 6.1

Cesarean Section w/o CC

DRG 372

MDC 14	RW$ 0.5534	Medical	Outlier Cutoff 9	Mean LOS 3.8

Vaginal Delivery with Complicating Diagnosis

DRG 373

MDC 14	RW$ 0.4063	Medical	Outlier Cutoff 9	Mean LOS 3.2

Vaginal Delivery w/o Complicating Diagnosis

MDC 14	RW$ 0.5492	Surgical	Outlier Cutoff 7	Mean LOS 3.6

Vaginal Delivery with Sterilization and/or D & C

MDC 14	RW$ 0.6889	Surgical	Outlier Cutoff 15	Mean LOS 4.4

Vaginal Delivery with Operating Room Procedures Except Sterilization and/or D & C

OPERATIVE PROCEDURES WITH POTENTIAL HOME CARE NEEDS

Hemorrhage control
Hemorrhoidectomy
Organ biopsy

MDC 14	RW$ 0.4158	Medical	Outlier Cutoff 10	Mean LOS 2.9

Postpartum Diagnoses w/o Operating Room Procedure

PRINCIPAL DIAGNOSES WITH POTENTIAL HOME CARE NEEDS

Postpartum complication
Viral disease, postpartum
Vaginal delivery laceration

MDC 14	RW$ 0.4761	Surgical	Outlier Cutoff 8	Mean LOS 2.2

Postpartum Diagnoses with Operating Room Procedure

OPERATIVE PROCEDURE WITH POTENTIAL HOME CARE NEEDS

Any operating room procedure for postpartum diagnosis

DRG 378

MDC 14	RW$ 0.8094	Medical	Outlier Cutoff 11	Mean LOS 5.5

Ectopic Pregnancy

DRG 379

MDC 14	RW$ 0.3169	Medical	Outlier Cutoff 8	Mean LOS 2.2

Threatened Abortion

PRINCIPAL DIAGNOSES WITH POTENTIAL HOME CARE NEEDS

Hemorrhage, early pregnancy
Threatened premature labor

DRG 380

MDC 14	RW$ 0.2705	Medical	Outlier Cutoff 4	Mean LOS 1.5

Abortion w/o D & C

PRINCIPAL DIAGNOSES WITH POTENTIAL HOME CARE NEEDS

Spontaneous abortion
Legal abortion
Illegal abortion with complications
Attempted abortion with complications

DRG 381

MDC 14	RW$ 0.3602	Medical	Outlier Cutoff 4	Mean LOS 1.4

Abortion with D & C

PRINCIPAL DIAGNOSES WITH POTENTIAL HOME CARE NEEDS

D & C for pregnancy termination
D & C postdelivery
Aspiration curettage for pregnancy termination

| MDC 14 | RW$ 0.1842 | Medical | Outlier Cutoff 2 | Mean LOS 1.2 |

False Labor

| MDC 14 | RW$ 0.4317 | Medical | Outlier Cutoff 14 | Mean LOS 3.4 |

Other Antepartum Diagnoses with Medical Complications

PRINCIPAL DIAGNOSES WITH POTENTIAL HOME CARE NEEDS

Infection
Hypertension
Abnormal glucose
Multiple delivery
Lactation complication
Drug dependence
Thrombophlebitis

| MDC 14 | RW$ 0.3245 | Medical | Outlier Cutoff 9 | Mean LOS 2.2 |

Other Antepartum Diagnoses w/o Medical Complications

PRINCIPAL DIAGNOSES WITH POTENTIAL HOME CARE NEEDS

Abnormality of birth canal
Abnormality of fetus
Prolonged labor

15 MDC 15
NEWBORNS AND OTHER NEONATES WITH CONDITIONS ORIGINATING IN THE PERINATAL PERIOD: NOS*

*NOS = not otherwise specified as Surgical or Medical (7 DRGs)

Neonates

Extreme Immaturity

Prematurity

Full-Term Neonate w/Major Problem

Neonates w/Significant Problems

Normal Newborns

Diagnoses in this MDC are usually treated on pediatric units or in pediatric hospitals. The follow-up care usually falls under maternal-child health programs in community agencies. Some diagnoses will need special follow-up care. The information and description in this MDC is included for completeness of the DRG listing, but the reader is referred to pediatric reference works for additional information.

DRG 385

MDC 15	RW$ 0.6883	No Specification	Outlier Cutoff 14	Mean LOS 1.8

Neonates, Died or Transferred

DRG 386

MDC 15	RW$ 3.6863	No Specification	Outlier Cutoff 38	Mean LOS 17.9

Extreme Immaturity, Neonate

DIAGNOSIS WITH POTENTIAL HOME CARE NEEDS

Extreme immaturity in neonate plus respiratory distress syndrome

DRG 387

MDC 15	RW$ 1.8459	No Specification	Outlier Cutoff 33	Mean LOS 13.3

Prematurity with Major Problems

(Need to identify major problems that would have long-term effect).

DRG 388

MDC 15	RW$ 1.1693	No Specification	Outlier Cutoff 29	Mean LOS 8.6

Prematurity w/o Major Problems

| MDC 15 | RW$ 0.5482 | No Specification | Outlier Cutoff 16 | Mean LOS 4.7 |

Full-Term Neonate with Major Problems

DIAGNOSES WITH POTENTIAL HOME CARE NEEDS

Birth defect
Birth trauma
Congenital defect

| MDC 15 | RW$ 0.3523 | No Specification | Outlier Cutoff 9 | Mean LOS 3.4 |

Neonates with Other Significant Problems

See **DRG 389.**

| MDC 15 | RW$ 0.2241 | No Specification | Outlier Cutoff 7 | Mean LOS 3.1 |

Normal Newborns

(Including multiple birth)

16 MDC 16
DISEASES AND DISORDERS OF BLOOD AND BLOOD-FORMING ORGANS

SURGICAL GROUPINGS (3 DRGs)

Splenectomy

MEDICAL GROUPINGS (5 DRGs)

Red Blood Cell Disorders

Coagulation Disorders

Reticuloendothelial and Immunity Disorders

MASTER HOME CARE PLANNING GUIDE FOR DISEASES AND DISORDERS OF BLOOD AND BLOOD-FORMING ORGANS

Pattern	Assessment Factor	Plan
1. Alteration in health management pattern	Assess effect of condition on patient's energy and stamina and ability to resist infection.	Give patient information on disease process. If the patient is highly susceptible to infection, teach isolation techniques for posthospital course. If patient is weak, instruct in progressive ambulation. See specific DRG.
2. Nutritional alteration	Assess patient's nutritional needs, especially in regard to vitamins and minerals such as iron. Also assess with regard to interaction of some medications with food substances.	Give patient detailed instructions in dietary changes or supplements that will be needed. See specific DRG.
3. Alteration in activity and exercise pattern	Assess patient's response of fatigue, joint or bone pain on ambulation and general activity. The underlying cause of some of the blood disorders may have more effect on the patient's activity than the diagnosis itself.	See specific DRG.
4. Knowledge deficit related to disease process and method of treatment	Assess patient/caregiver's ability to comprehend plan of therapy. Determine from the physician the plan of care following discharge.	Instruct patient in the plan. Assist in locating community resources for special medications, lab work or procedures. See specific DRG.
5. Alteration in self-concept secondary to anxiety regarding long-term effect of diagnosis	Assess patient/caregiver's ability to understand diagnosis and potential long-term effect.	See specific DRG.
6. Alteration in role-relationship pattern.	Assess effect of high susceptibility on social isolation for long periods of time. Assess potential effect on family interaction and/or normal social development.	See specific DRG.

MDC 16	RW$ 2.7746	Surgical	Outlier Cutoff 36	Mean LOS 16.4

Splenectomy – Age $\geq$ 18

OPERATIVE PROCEDURES WITH POTENTIAL HOME CARE NEEDS

Partial and total splenectomy
Repair of spleen

DETAILS TO CONSIDER

Some splenectomies are done as a result of trauma or splenic disease, and some are done as a therapy for a blood disorder. The follow-up needs will depend on the reason for the splenectomy.

POTENTIAL HOME CARE PROBLEMS

PLAN

1. Health management deficit secondary to medical diagnosis.

Determine extent of patient's medical problems and instruct patient in aspects of the disease. If the patient is over 65, assess impact of surgery and diagnosis on patient's ability to care for self. Also assess availability and ability of caregiver.

1a. Potential for postoperative infection.

Instruct patient in signs and symptoms of infection and to call physician immediately if symptoms occur. If patient might have difficulty obtaining antibiotics in a short time because of lack of transportation or distant pharmacy, have patient obtain a prescription and have the medication available in the home. Quick institution of antibiotic therapy is important.

1b. Potential for postoperative respiratory complication, especially pneumonia.

Instruct patient to continue respiratory exercises at home, to avoid smoking or being around smoke and to avoid contact with persons with respiratory illness. Some physicians recommend Pneumovax (pneumococcal vaccine) as a protection for the patient.

1c. Potential for delayed postoperative formation of bilirubin gallstones.

Check with the patient's physician to determine relationship of diagnosis to gallstone formation. If appropriate, instruct patient to observe for signs and symptoms of gallstone formation such as substernal pain, change in stool color or discomfort after eating fatty foods.

2. Alteration in activity/exercise pattern.

Assess patient's ability to do activities of daily living. There may be a gradual improvement in the patient's health status over a period of 3–5 months.

REFERRAL INFORMATION

Unless the patient is elderly or has other complications he/she should need minimal assistance. Referral for follow-up monitoring of disease progression and for signs/symptoms of complications is indicated.

DRG 393

MDC 16	RW$ 1.5366	Surgical	Outlier Cutoff 29	Mean LOS 9.1

Splenectomy – Age 0–17

OPERATIVE PROCEDURES WITH POTENTIAL HOME CARE NEEDS

See **DRG 392.**

DETAILS TO CONSIDER

The reader is encouraged to consult pediatric references for additional information.

DRG 394

MDC 16	RW$ 1.1146	Surgical	Outlier Cutoff 26	Mean LOS 6.1

Other Operating Room Procedures of the Blood and Blood-Forming Organs

OPERATIVE PROCEDURES WITH POTENTIAL HOME CARE NEEDS

Thymus operation
Exploratory laparotomy

DETAILS TO CONSIDER

Procedures in this diagnostic group are done to determine the stage of a disease or, as in the case of thymus operation, as a treatment. The long-term needs of the patient will be directly affected by the findings of the staging procedure. Needs vary greatly from stage to stage. The reader is referred to texts on hematology and oncology for further information.

Red Blood Cell Disorders – Age $> = 18$

DIAGNOSES WITH POTENTIAL HOME CARE NEEDS

Anemia
Sickle cell anemia
Aplastic anemia

DETAILS TO CONSIDER

These conditions are chronic, and the patient admitted to an acute care hospital with these diagnoses are usually admitted for a complication of the disease. Long-term needs are great in chronic diseases and follow-up medical care is vital.

POTENTIAL HOME CARE PROBLEMS

1. Health management deficit secondary to long-term disease.

1a. Potential for infection.

2. Potential for ineffective coping.

PLAN

Assess patient's knowledge of disease process and course of illness. Assess patient's/caregiver's ability to manage care.

Instruct patient in signs/symptoms of infection, especially hepatitis in patients who receive transfusions.

Plans for counseling of patients and families of patients with sickle cell disease should be made. Problems needing long-term counseling include pain control with potential for narcotic addiction, potential for depression and the need for genetic counseling.

REFERRAL INFORMATION

A referral to a home health agency and/or mental health agency should be made for patients and families of patients with sickle cell anemia.

Red Blood Cell Disorders – Age 0–17

DIAGNOSES WITH POTENTIAL HOME CARE NEEDS

Same as **DRG 395.**

DETAILS TO CONSIDER

The reader is referred to pediatric references for more information.

DRG 397

MDC 16   **RW$ 0.9863**   **Medical**   **Outlier Cutoff 27**   **Mean LOS 6.7**

Coagulation Disorders

DIAGNOSES WITH POTENTIAL HOME CARE NEEDS

Congenital factor disorder
Coagulation deficiency
Thrombocytopenia
Hemorrhagic conditions

DETAILS TO CONSIDER

The conditions can be life-threatening and can lead to complications. Since conditions in this DRG can occur in the young, the reader is also referred to pediatric references for additional information.

POTENTIAL HOME CARE PROBLEMS

1. Health management deficit secondary to treatment for coagulation disorder.

2. Alteration in activity/exercise secondary to joint involvement.

PLAN

The hemophiliac patient and family should be provided intense education so that the institution of therapy can be started at home at the first sign of bleeding. Education needs include management of self-venipuncture, administration of IV therapy factor, dose selection, early recognition of problems and activities to prevent bleeding episodes. Since some coagulation disorders are acquired, such as malabsorption of Vitamin K, effects of anticoagulant therapy and liver disease, the educational needs will vary depending on the cause.

Assess the patient's joint disease status. In some patients joint disease may interfere with ability to carry out activities of daily living. The knees, ankles, elbows, hips and shoulders may be involved and there may be major long-term disability.

REFERRAL INFORMATION

Referral of patient and family to a hemophilia center should be made since the educational needs of this condition are many. The impact of these conditions on the patient's social interactions, job setting and self-care need to be addressed on a long-term basis. Local medical and laboratory follow-up must be arranged so that the patient can have easy access to therapy. The use of an emergency warning bracelet should be encouraged.

MDC 16   RW$ 0.8900   Medical   Outlier Cutoff 26   Mean LOS 6.1

Reticuloendothelial and Immunity Disorders
Age > = 70 and/or CC

DIAGNOSES WITH POTENTIAL HOME CARE NEEDS

Blood diseases
Immune mechanism disease, including AIDS (Acquired Immune Deficiency Syndrome)

DETAILS TO CONSIDER

The reticuloendothelial system is more a functional system than an anatomical one, and it functions as an important defense mechanism. Patients with disease in this group are generally admitted to the hospital because of a complication of the disease. Therefore the number of admissions to this DRG is relatively small. These diagnoses would be considered the secondary diagnosis.

One of the diseases in this group is AIDS which can pose a challenge to the discharge planner. The disease manifestations include many opportunistic infections such as pneumo, cytomegalovirus and anogenital herpes. The U.S. Center for Disease Control has published isolation recommendations, including strict precautions for clinical staff, to avoid contact of skin, mucous membranes, blood, blood products, excretions, secretions and tissue of suspected cases. There is a prolonged incubation and the status of the carrier state is unknown. Patients with AIDS can either be treated in a hospital or in the home.

POTENTIAL HOME CARE PROBLEMS

PLAN

1. Health management deficit secondary to overwhelming illness and guarded prognosis.

Interview family members or significant others to determine ability to manage care of the patient. Determine the level of care needed related to severity of symptoms and the response to treatment.

1a. Susceptibility to infection.

The patient will not only be isolated to protect the caregiver, but to protect the patient. The hallmark of this disease is that it suppresses immunity to infection.

2. Altered nutrition.

Do nutritional assessment and determine need for IV fluid and nutritional supplements.

3. Alteration in elimination.

In patients with anogenital herpes there is special need for post-voiding and bowel movement hygiene. Pain control is vital!

4. Alteration in activity tolerance.

In latter stages of these diseases the patient becomes too weak to ambulate. Arrangement should be made for ambulation assistive devices and skin comfort measures while the patient is in bed.

5. Cognitive alteration.

In some patients the disease process affects the nervous system and the patient may have seizure activity. This information must be communicated to family and home care staff so that a safe environment can be provided.

6. Alteration in role-relationship.

The clinical need to isolate patients and the fear of the disease contribute to social isolation. The long-term sensory deprivation may be difficult to handle for the patient and family. Counseling may be necessary.

7. Ineffective family coping.

This rare diagnosis is very difficult for some families to accept because of the homosexual and drug-use implications. Counseling by a medical/social worker is vital for family stability.

REFERRAL INFORMATION

The referral must include all the diagnoses and complications. The plan for isolation technique must be made prior to the patient's discharge. The patient may require IV fluids and medications at home which can also pose an isolation problem. Early referral is important so that staff selection and training can be carried out. Refer to DRGs discussing other diagnoses the patient may have.

DRG 399

MDC 16	RW$ 0.8459	Medical	Outlier Cutoff 26	Mean LOS 5.6

Reticuloendothelial and Immunity Disorders – Age < 70 w/o CC

See **DRG 398.**

17 MDC 17 MYELOPROLIFERATIVE DISORDERS

SURGICAL GROUPINGS (6 DRGs)

Lymphoma or Leukemia

Myeloproliferative Disorders

Poorly Differentiated Neoplasm

MEDICAL GROUPINGS (9 DRGs)

Lymphoma or Leukemia

Radiotherapy

Chemotherapy

History of Malignancy with or w/o Endoscopy

Other Myeloproliferative Disorders

Poorly Differentiated Neoplasm

MASTER HOME CARE PLANNING GUIDE
FOR MYELOPROLIFERATIVE DISORDERS

Pattern	Assessment Factors	Plan
1. Health management deficit secondary to potential for infection	Does the patient's blood cell count put him/her at great risk for infection? Is the patient in remission? Does the patient need reverse isolation to protect him/her from exposure to life-threatening infections?	Instruct patient, family and friends of need to prevent exposure to ill persons if the blood count indicates this need.
2. Alteration in nutrition secondary to diagnosis and treatment	What is the nutritional state of the patient? Is the patient cachexic? What is the extent of organ system involvement? Is an anorexia pattern associated with systemic effects of treatment? Does oral pain as a consequence of therapy interfere with the patient's ability to take nourishment? Have surgery, chemotherapy and radiotherapy had a cumulative effect on the patient's nutritional reserves?	Have a nutritional consult to determine needs and method of supplementing those needs, including consideration of the need for TPN (Total Parental Nutrition) or enteral feeding through a tube.
3. Alteration in elimination	Does therapy prescribed leave the patient with an increased risk of hyperuricemia? Do the effects of therapy include diarrhea and lead to fluid and electrolyte depletion? Does the nutritional support plan have effect on bowel pattern such as constipation or diarrhea? Does the patient have anal fistulae that need to be treated?	Interview patient for signs and symptoms of problems that may be treated with medications or changes in nutritional supply. Instruct patient and family for need to monitor output and inform physician of changes.
4. Alteration in activity and exercise pattern secondary to malaise and fatigue from disease process and/or therapy.	What activities can the patient manage alone and what type of assistance is needed? Can patient bathe or eat independently? What are the long-term expectations in energy level? Is the patient prone to decubiti or contracture because of the need for bedrest? Will the patient need assistance in transportation for daily or weekly outpatient therapy? Can he/she sit in a car for the trip or is an ambulance required?	Involve physical therapy for an assessment and plan for ambulation. Instruct family in measures to prevent adverse effects of bedrest. Assist family in making arrangements for transportation to and from therapy sessions.
5. Alteration in cognitive pattern **5a.** secondary to pain management	What is effective for relief of pain for the patient? Does he/she require scheduled narcotics? Is IV morphine required? Has the patient had surgery, radiotherapy or chemotherapy to control pain? Can topical agents control oral pain?	Evaluate all aspects of pain and consult with physician and pharmacist to work out a plan for control of pain. Instruct patient and family in the plan for pain control and in the fact that the plan can vary after discharge according to the changing needs of the patient.

5b. secondary to central nervous system involvement	What are the sensory effects of the disease? Is the patient confused or reacting to normal effects of pain medication? Has the patient had a cerebral infarction or brain involvement?	Instruct family in the fact that behavior changes are not uncommon and that they are sometimes the most difficult thing for the family members to endure. Instruct them in early signs of CNS problems and to communicate those problems early.
6. Sleep-rest pattern interruption	Does the patient sleep for prolonged periods? Will the caregiver have an opportunity to sleep? Do changes need to be made in sleeping arrangements at home, such as converting a family room to a bedroom for the patient?	Discuss sleeping arrangements and help patient and family make decisions about home set-up. Give patient sources for home equipment and supplies so that arrangements can be made and set up prior to discharge.
7. Alteration in self-concept and anxiety secondary to guarded diagnosis	Determine patient/family ability to understand diagnosis and prognosis. Is the patient or family severely depressed and so fearful that they have difficulty coping with everyday life functions?	Consult with medical and social worker and oncology clinicians to determine long-term needs. If necessary request psychiatric evaluation and treatment.
8. Alteration in role-relation secondary to interruption in parenting, role reversal or social isolation	Does the patient have young children who will need counseling? Will the patient be able to continue in parenting role? Will the patient be able to work? Is the patient now dependent where he/she used to be independent?	Refer for counseling as stated above.

REFERRAL INFORMATION

Patients with diagnoses in this MDC should be referred to a hospice unit. There are various types of units including inpatient for therapy or respite care. There are hospice units in home health agencies that offer a variety of services and a variety of resources. A referral to a hospice unit is appropriate no matter what the stage of illness or length of time projected before the patient is terminal. Establishing rapport and early intervention is valuable for the patient and family and hospice resources may be used minimally at first. The definition of terminal hospice care of about six months duration is a general rule. For families and patients who go into remission the support of the hospice team, including nurses, physicians, medical social workers, pharmacists, pastoral counselors, volunteers and home health aides is invaluable.

An initial investigation of financial resources should be started by the family while the patient is still hospitalized. The family needs to address finances early and needs to be encouraged to do so. Some families may feel guilty and wish to do anything, no matter what the cost and others will feel overwhelmed. Preplanning will help in selection of necessary services and equipment in a timely and cost effective manner.

DRG 400

MDC 17	RW$ 2.8272	Surgical	Outlier Cutoff 37	Mean LOS 16.9

Lymphoma or Leukemia with Major Operating Room Procedure

OPERATIVE PROCEDURE WITH POTENTIAL HOME CARE NEEDS

Lymphoma or leukemia with major operating room procedure

DETAILS TO CONSIDER

The long-term needs will depend on the operative procedure and the stage of illness. Refer to the DRG discussing the OR procedure.

POTENTIAL HOME CARE PROBLEMS	PLAN
1. Health management deficit secondary to high risk of wound infection or post-op complications.	Instruct patient in care of the wound and in signs and symptoms of infection.
2. Alteration in activity/exercise with self-care deficit.	Assess impact of need for prolonged recuperation from surgery on patient's ability to care for self.

DRG 401

MDC 17	RW$ 1.2409	Surgical	Outlier Cutoff 29	Mean LOS 8.9

Lymphoma or Leukemia with Minor Operating Room Procedures – Age > = 70 and/or CC

See **DRG 400.**

DRG 402

MDC 17	RW$ 1.1316	Surgical	Outlier Cutoff 27	Mean LOS 7.1

Lymphoma or Leukemia with Minor Operating Room Procedure – Age < 70 w/o CC

See **DRG 400.**

MDC 17   RW$ 1.1715   Medical   Outlier Cutoff 27   Mean LOS 7.1

Lymphoma or Leukemia – Age > = 70 and/or CC

DIAGNOSES WITH POTENTIAL HOME CARE NEEDS

Lymphoma or leukemia

DETAILS TO CONSIDER

Method of treatment and ability of patient to receive therapy as an outpatient will affect long-term needs.

POTENTIAL HOME CARE PROBLEM

Health care deficit secondary to need for long-term and complex therapy.

PLAN

Instruct patient and family in disease process and planned medical follow-up.

REFERRAL INFORMATION

Elderly patients tolerate therapy poorly and have a decreased chance for remission. The patient may have increased needs as the disease progresses.

MDC 17   RW$ 1.1787   Medical   Outlier Cutoff 26   Mean LOS 6.4

Lymphoma or Leukemia – Age 18–69 w/o CC

Same as **DRG 403.**

MDC 17   RW$ 1.0517   Medical   Outlier Cutoff 25   Mean LOS 4.9

Lymphoma or Leukemia – Age 0–17

Same as **DRG 403.**

DETAILS TO CONSIDER

The reader is referred to pediatric references for additional information.

DRG 406

MDC 17	RW$ 2.2671	Surgical	Outlier Cutoff 35	Mean LOS 15.0

Myeloproliferative Disorders or Poorly Differentiated Neoplasm with Major Operating Room Procedures and CC

See DRG 400.

DRG 407

MDC 17	RW$ 2.1366	Surgical	Outlier Cutoff 33	Mean LOS 13.3

Myeloproliferative Disorders or Poorly Differentiated Neoplasm with Major Operating Room Procedures w/o CC

See DRG 400.

DRG 408

MDC 17	RW$ 1.1389	Surgical	Outlier Cutoff 27	Mean LOS 7.1

Myeloproliferative Disorders or Poorly Differentiated Neoplasm with Minor Operating Room Procedures

See DRG 400.

MDC 17   **RW\$ 0.8134**   **Medical**   **Outlier Cutoff 26**   **Mean LOS 5.7**

Radiotherapy

DIAGNOSTIC PROCEDURES WITH POTENTIAL HOME CARE NEEDS

Radiotherapy session.
Radiotherapy follow-up

DETAILS TO CONSIDER

Long-term needs will depend on the underlying diagnosis and reason for radiation therapy. It will also depend on the organ or organs involved, the functioning of those organs and structures adjacent to the part being irradiated. Refer to the MDC discussing the system involved. In some cases the patient is admitted for radiotherapy because of the distance the patient lives from the therapy center.

POTENTIAL HOME CARE PPROBLEMS

PLAN

1. Health management deficit secondary to side effects of radiotherapy.

Have patient be aware of possible side effects such as nausea, vomiting, mucous membrane inflammation, pneumonitis and dermatitis. Be sure patient has adequate medications to relieve these symptoms.

2. Alteration in activity secondary to radiotherapy.

If side effects will decrease patient's ability to carry out activities of daily living additional home health services should be considered.

REFERRAL INFORMATION

See **DRG 410.**

DRG 410

MDC 17   **RW$ 0.3527**   **Medical**   **Outlier Cutoff 12**   **Mean LOS 2.6**

Chemotherapy

DIAGNOSTIC PROCEDURES WITH POTENTIAL HOME CARE NEEDS
Maintenance chemotherapy
Chemotherapy follow-up

DETAILS TO CONSIDER
Long-term needs will depend on the underlying diagnosis and reason for chemotherapy. If the therapy is aimed at palliation, the dose of the chemotherapeutic agent may be prescribed at a level which will not cause many side effects. If a cure is the aim, the dosage level may cause transient side effects that need intervention. The patient may be admitted for a diagnostic study which cannot be done as an outpatient or may be admitted for a chemotherapy treatment with a planned pretreatment protocol such as for cisplatin.

POTENTIAL HOME CARE PROBLEMS

PLAN

1. Health management deficit secondary to side effects of chemotherapy.

Have patient aware of possible systemic side effects of therapy including fatigue, weakness, nausea, vomiting, mucous membrane involvement and loss of hair. Preventive measures can be taken to alleviate known side effects of the medication.

2. Alteration in activity/exercise pattern secondary to chemotherapy.

If side effects of therapy will decrease patient's ability to carry out activities of daily living, the need for additional home health services should be considered.

REFERRAL INFORMATION
Since this is a short-term admission the preadmission home care services need to be evaluated in relation to the effect of chemotherapy. If side effects are expected that will decrease the patient's ability to carry out activities of daily living, additional home care services should be considered. For continuity of care, the agency providing home health services prior to admission, if any, should be contacted and given current clinical information.

MDC 17   **RW$ 0.7221**   **Medical**   **Outlier Cutoff 25**   **Mean LOS 4.7**

History of Malignancy w/o Endoscopy

DIAGNOSTIC PROCEDURES WITH POTENTIAL HOME CARE NEEDS

Malignancy of various body organs
Diagnostic work-up other than endoscopy

DETAILS TO CONSIDER

This is a rarely used DRG since most admissions for patients with malignancy are classified with the type of malignancy.* The long-term needs will depend on the outcome of the diagnostic work-up. Refer to DRGs discussing the related diagnosis.

*Many diagnostic work-ups are done as outpatient procedures and only as inpatient procedures if they have complicated post-study monitoring or the patient is symptomatic.

MDC 17   **RW$ 0.3400**   **Medical**   **Outlier Cutoff 8**   **Mean LOS 2.0**

History of Malignancy with Endoscopy

DIAGNOSTIC PROCEDURE WITH POTENTIAL HOME CARE NEEDS

Diagnostic work-up including endoscopy

DETAILS TO CONSIDER

See **DRG 411.**

The postendoscopy monitoring depends on the organ or organs being endoscoped. Types of endoscopy include such procedures as; bronchoscopy (for lung conditions), ERCP or endoscopic retrograde cholangiopancreatography (for conditions of the biliary tract), gastroscopy (for conditions of the stomach), sigmoidoscopy (for conditions of the rectum and sigmoid colon) and cystoscopy (for conditions of the urinary tract).

Note that length of stay for patients having endoscopy is shorter than those not having endoscopy.

DRG 413

MDC 17	RW$ 1.0975	Medical	Outlier Cutoff 27	Mean LOS 7.3

Other Myeloprolific Disorders or
Poorly Differentiated Neoplasm Diagnosis – Age > = 70 and/or CC

DIAGNOSES WITH POTENTIAL HOME CARE NEEDS

Cancer in situ
Benign neoplasm

DETAILS TO CONSIDER

The malignancy in this DRG is in situ which means it is confined to the primary site. The long-term needs will depend on the site involved and the choice of medical management. Refer to DRGs discussing the system in which the organ involved is discussed.

DRG 414

MDC 17	RW$ 1.0359	Medical	Outlier Cutoff 26	Mean LOS 6.4

Other Myeloprolific Disorders or
Poorly Differentiated Neoplasm Diagnosis – Age < 70 w/o CC

DIAGNOSES WITH POTENTIAL HOME CARE NEEDS

Cancer in situ
Benign neoplasm

DETAILS TO CONSIDER

See DRG 413.

18 MDC 18
INFECTIOUS AND PARASITIC DISEASES

SURGICAL GROUPINGS (1 DRG)

Operating Room Procedures

MEDICAL GROUPINGS (8 DRGs)

Septicemia

Postoperative and Posttraumatic Infections

Fever of Unknown Origin

Viral Illness

MASTER HOME CARE PLANNING GUIDE
FOR INFECTIOUS AND PARASITIC DISEASES

Pattern	Assessment Factors	Plan
1. Health management deficit secondary to infection	Determination of the infectious disease clinical course, method of transmission and susceptible hosts must be done to determine follow-up care. In cases where there is a wound infection, determine patient and caregiver's ability to care for the wound.	See specific DRG. Use references on infectious diseases for more information on specific agent.
2. Alteration in nutrition secondary to infection	Assess patient's nutritional fluid needs and additional caloric needs during healing and recovery.	Consult with physician and dietition. Instruct patient and caregiver in nutritional needs and methods to meet those needs.
3. Activity/exercise tolerance	Assess patient's ability to increase ambulation and self-care following resolution of infection.	If patient has limitations in ambulation because of decreased tolerance or prolonged bedrest, initiate physical therapy. If patient is unable to do self-care at time of discharge a home health aide will be needed for personal care.
4. Alteration in role-relationship secondary to need for isolation for infectious disease	Determine type and length of isolation indicated for each disease.	Instruct patient/family in isolation protocol for the various agents.

DRG 415

MDC 18	RW$ 3.0027	Surgical	Outlier Cutoff 35	Mean LOS 15.1

Operating Room Procedures for Infectious and Parasitic Diseases

OPERATIVE PROCEDURES WITH POTENTIAL HOME CARE NEEDS

Any operating room procedures with principal diagnosis of infection or parasitic disease.

DETAILS TO CONSIDER

The long-term needs will depend on the procedure and the specific disease. Refer to DRGs that cover the specific surgical procedure or disease.

MDC 18	RW$ 1.5504	Medical	Outlier Cutoff 29	Mean LOS 9.2

Septicemia – Age > = 18

DIAGNOSES WITH POTENTIAL HOME CARE NEEDS

Bacteremia
Septicemia NEC and NOS

DETAILS TO CONSIDER

Long-term needs will depend on the clinical effect of the disease, the organs involved and the effect of the disease on the functions of that organ or system. For example, if the septicemia is related to meningococcus, there may be substantial sequelae that need long-term care. See MDCs related to the system involved for further information.

MDC 18	RW$ 0.7152	Medical	Outlier Cutoff 20	Mean LOS 5.2

Septicemia – Age 0–17

Same as **DRG 416.**

DETAILS TO CONSIDER

The reader is referred to pediatric references for more information.

MDC 18	RW$ 0.9968	Medical	Outlier Cutoff 28	Mean LOS 8.4

Postoperative and Posttraumatic Infections

DIAGNOSES WITH POTENTIAL HOME CARE NEEDS

Postoperative and posttraumatic infections

DETAILS TO CONSIDER

Some patients in this DRG will have an open wound and some may have an osteomyelitis. The patient will have gone to the operating room on this admission since this is a Medical DRG.

POTENTIAL HOME CARE PROBLEMS

1. Health maintenance deficit related to type of posthospital therapy.

1a. Long-term IV antibiotic therapy.

1b. Posthospital need for wound care.

PLAN

Determine plans for medical management.

If patient is a candidate for long-term IV therapy consult with the IV therapist and infectious disease physician to determine appropriate method of therapy. Medication can be self-administered at home with site changes done in the home by a home IV therapy nurse or in an outpatient setting. Assessment of the ability of the patient to carry out the therapy is the most important part of this method of therapy.

If the patient will need wound care, assess the degree of difficulty of the wound care for the patient. If the site is easy to reach and requires a simple dressing, teach the patient and family how to do the dressing. If the wound is not easy to reach or needs to be irrigated with a catheter or needs to be packed, refer to a home health agency for skilled nursing visits.

DRG 419

MDC 18	RW$ 0.8628	Medical	Outlier Cutoff 27	Mean LOS 6.9

Fever of Unknown Origin – Age > = 70 and/or CC

DIAGNOSIS WITH POTENTIAL HOME CARE NEEDS

Fever of unknown origin

DETAILS TO CONSIDER

The long-term needs will depend on the effect of the fever on the patient's ability to carry out activities of daily living and the secondary diagnosis. Refer to DRGs that discuss the secondary diagnosis if it is known.

DRG 420

MDC 18	RW$ 0.8022	Medical	Outlier Cutoff 26	Mean LOS 6.2

Fever of Unknown Origin – Age 18–69 w/o CC

Fever of unknown origin

See **DRG 419.**

MDC 18	RW$ 0.6045	Medical	Outlier Cutoff 21	Mean LOS 5.4

Viral Illness – Age $> = 18$

DIAGNOSIS WITH POTENTIAL HOME CARE NEEDS

Viral illness

DETAILS TO CONSIDER

The long-term needs of the patient will depend on the clinical effect of the viral illness and the patient's ability to carry out activities of daily living.

MDC 18	RW$ 0.4360	Medical	Outlier Cutoff 10	Mean LOS 3.2

Viral Illness and Fever of Unknown Origin – Age 0–17

DIAGNOSES WITH POTENTIAL HOME CARE NEEDS

Viral illness and fever of unknown origin

DETAILS TO CONSIDER

The reader is referred to pediatric references for more information.

MDC 18	RW$ 1.2107	Medical	Outlier Cutoff 29	Mean LOS 8.8

Other Infectious and Parasitic Disease Diagnoses

DIAGNOSES WITH POTENTIAL HOME CARE NEEDS

Other infectious and parasitic disease diagnoses

DETAILS TO CONSIDER

Diagnoses in this category include admission for the treatment of various infections or parasitic diseases. The long-term needs will depend on the clinical effect of the illness and the method of therapy. This DRG can include all age groups. The reader is referred to pediatric references if additional information is needed.

19 MDC 19
MENTAL DISEASES AND DISORDERS

SURGICAL GROUPINGS (1 DRG)

Operating Room Procedures

MEDICAL GROUPINGS (8 DRGs)

Acute Adjustment Reactions

Depressive Neuroses

Neuroses

Disorders of Personality and Impulse Control

Organic Disturbances and Mental Retardation

Psychoses

Childhood Mental Disorders

Diagnoses in this MDC are usually treated in specialty hospitals or institutes. The follow-up care falls under mental health programs. Some diagnoses will need follow-up care separate from mental health but those diagnoses are covered under other DRGs. The information and description in this MDC is included for the completeness of the DRG listing. The reader is referred to mental health and psychiatric references for additional information. At the time of the preparation of this book, psychiatric units and hospitals were not under the Medicare Prospective Payment System which utilizes DRGs.

DRG 424

MDC 19	RW$ 2.1938	Surgical	Outlier Cutoff 34	Mean LOS 14.2

Operating Room Procedures with Principal Diagnosis of Mental Illness

DRG 425

MDC 19	RW$ 0.6812	Medical	Outlier Cutoff 26	Mean LOS 5.8

Acute Adjustment Reaction and Disturbances of Psychosocial Dysfunction

Antisocial behavior
Delirium
Anxiety state
Stress reaction
Hallucinations
Psychogenic fugue

DRG 426

MDC 19	RW$ 0.9495	Medical	Outlier Cutoff 29	Mean LOS 9.4

Depressive Neuroses

| MDC 19 | RW$ 0.7678 | Medical | Outlier Cutoff 27 | Mean LOS 6.9 |

Neuroses Except Depressive

Phobiae
Neurotic disorders
Adjustment reaction

| MDC 19 | RW$ 0.9741 | Medical | Outlier Cutoff 28 | Mean LOS 8.3 |

Disorders of Personality and Impulse Control

| MDC 19 | RW$ 0.9523 | Medical | Outlier Cutoff 29 | Mean LOS 8.8 |

Organic Disturbances and Mental Retardation

Organic brain syndrome
Retardation

| MDC 19 | RW$ 1.0934 | Medical | Outlier Cutoff 31 | Mean LOS 10.8 |

Psychoses

DRG 431

MDC 19　　**RW$ 2.2519**　　**Medical**　　**Outlier Cutoff 35**　　**Mean LOS 15.4**

Childhood Mental Disorders

Pica
Enuresis
Encopresis
Relationship problems
Pyromania
Emotional disorder

DRG 432

MDC 19　　**RW$ 1.0525**　　**Medical**　　**Outlier Cutoff 27**　　**Mean LOS 7.2**

Other Diagnoses of Mental Disorders

Psychosexual dysfunction
Eating disorder (nonorganic)
Sleeping disturbance

20 MDC 20
SUBSTANCE USE AND
SUBSTANCE-INDUCED
ORGANIC MENTAL DISORDERS: NOS*

***NOS = not otherwise specified as
Surgical or Medical (6 DRGs)**

Left Against Medical Advice

Drug Dependence

Alcohol Dependence

Alcohol and Substance-Induced
Organic Mental Syndrome

Diagnoses in this MDC are usually treated in specialty hospitals or institutions. The follow-up care falls under mental health, drug and alcohol abuse and dependency programs. The information and description in this MDC is included for the completeness of the DRG listing. The reader is referred to mental health, psychiatric, drug and alcohol dependency references.

DRG 433

MDC 20	RW$ 0.4457	No Specification	Outlier Cutoff 17	Mean LOS 2.5

Substance Use and Substance-Induced Organic Mental Disorders, Left Against Medical Advice

DRG 434

MDC 20	RW$ 1.0404	No Specification	Outlier Cutoff 29	Mean LOS 9.1

Drug Dependence

DRG 435

MDC 20	RW$ 1.0738	No Specification	Outlier Cutoff 28	Mean LOS 8.0

Drug Use Except Dependence

Drug abuse, episodic, in remission

DRG 436

MDC 20	RW$ 0.8853	No Specification	Outlier Cutoff 28	Mean LOS 8.1

Alcohol Dependence

| MDC 20 | RW$ 0.6183 | No Specification | Outlier Cutoff 24 | Mean LOS 3.5 |

Alcohol Use Except Dependence

Alcohol abuse, episodic or in remission

| MDC 20 | RW$ 0.8420 | No Specification | Outlier Cutoff 27 | Mean LOS 6.9 |

Alcohol and Substance-Induced Organic Mental Syndrome

Delirium tremens
Alcoholic psychosis
Drug-induced mental disorder

21 MDC 21
INJURIES, POISONINGS AND TOXIC EFFECT OF DRUGS

SURGICAL GROUPINGS (5 DRGs)

Skin Grafts

Wound Debridements

Hand Procedures

MEDICAL GROUPINGS (12 DRGs)

Multiple Trauma

Allergic Reactions

Toxic Effects of Drugs

Complications of Treatment

MASTER CARE PLANNING GUIDE
FOR INJURIES, POISONINGS, AND TOXIC EFFECTS OF DRUGS

Pattern	Assessment Factor	Plan
1. Health management deficit secondary to trauma or traumatic experience	What were the circumstances of the injury and what is the impact on the patient and family?	Determine patient's ability to care for self and interview family. If the patient is elderly and lives alone, assess the safety of this arrangement. If there is suspicion of intentional maltreatment report to the proper authorities.
2. Alteration in skin integrity	If the injury is thermal related or a drug reaction assess the effect on the skin, especially in situations in which future breakdown is possible.	Evaluate patient's skin condition and be sure patient has adequate warm clothing and a warm environment, adequate nutrition and fluids.
3. Alteration in activity and exercise	Assess patient's ability to carry out activities of daily living, especially if hands are involved, or if patient is confused. Assess patient's ability to ambulate safely.	See specific DRG.
3a. Potential for home maintenance management	If the patient lives alone or lives with another ill or elderly person, or is the caregiver to another ill person, assessment of the safety of this situation must be made.	Conduct a multidisciplinary conference including such persons as the physician, nursing staff, social service, occupational and physical therapist, pharmacist and family if possible to discuss long-term plans.
4. Alteration in cognitive thought processes	Evaluate sensory deficit and changes in thought process to determine if the changes are due to toxic effect or injury of if the injury resulted from a thought process deficit such as confusion.	Include discussion about patient behavior and thought process in above mentioned conference.

| MDC 21 | RW$ 1.8219 | Surgical | Outlier Cutoff 29 | Mean LOS 8.9 |

Skin Grafts for Injuries

OPERATIVE PROCEDURES WITH POTENTIAL HOME CARE NEEDS

Skin grafts for injuries

DETAILS TO CONSIDER

Skin grafting is a procedure usually done after the patient has been stabilized and may even be done during subsequent admissions. In some cases there may be more than one admission for skin grafting. The long-term needs will depend on the site of the injury and the effect on the patient's ability to carry out activities of daily living and do wound care.

See **Master Care Plan** for **MDC 22.**

POTENTIAL HOME CARE PROBLEM	PLAN
Health management deficit secondary to graft site and donor site management.	Instruct patient and caregiver in procedures for care of wounds.

| MDC 21 | RW$ 1.4807 | Surgical | Outlier Cutoff 27 | Mean LOS 7.2 |

Wound Debridement for Injuries

OPERATIVE PROCEDURE WITH POTENTIAL HOME CARE NEEDS

Wound debridement for injuries

DETAILS TO CONSIDER

Long-term needs will depend on the site and extent of the wound. The plan for method of healing such as by secondary granulation or by future skin grafting will have impact on the plan.

See **Master Care Plan** for **MDC 22.**

DRG 441

| MDC 21 | RW$ 0.7180 | Surgical | Outlier Cutoff 16 | Mean LOS 3.0 |

Hand Procedures for Injuries

OPERATIVE PROCEDURES WITH POTENTIAL HOME CARE NEEDS

Hand procedures for injuries

DETAILS TO CONSIDER

If both hands or if the dominant hand of the patient are involved the patient will have more needs.

POTENTIAL HOME CARE PROBLEM

Health management deficit secondary to injury.

PLAN

Refer for occupational therapy as soon as patient is stable. Patient will need to learn how to carry out activities of daily living with one hand or with both hands injured.

REFERRAL INFORMATION

Unless the patient has other medical problems, he/she should be able to receive occupational therapy on an outpatient basis.

DRG 442

| MDC 21 | RW$ 1.9026 | Surgical | Outlier Cutoff 29 | Mean LOS 9.1 |

Other Operating Room Procedures for Injuries
Age $>=$ 70 and/or CC

OPERATIVE PROCEDURES WITH POTENTIAL HOME CARE NEEDS

Other operating room procedures for injuries

DETAILS TO CONSIDER

This DRG is used when the injury cannot be classified under a more specific group such as a hip fracture or burns; therefore the long-term need will depend on the part of the body involved and the patient's ability to carry out activities of daily living.

| MDC 21 | RW$ 1.5211 | Surgical | Outlier Cutoff 27 | Mean LOS 6.6 |

Other Operating Room Procedures for Injuries – Age < 70 w/o CC

OPERATIVE PROCEDURES WITH POTENTIAL HOME CARE NEEDS

Other operating room procedures for injuries

See **DRG 442.**

| MDC 21 | RW$ 0.8830 | Medical | Outlier Cutoff 27 | Mean LOS 6.7 |

Multiple Trauma – Age > = 70 and/or CC

DIAGNOSIS WITH POTENTIAL HOME CARE NEEDS

Multiple trauma

DETAILS TO CONSIDER

Patients listed in this DRG have multiple injuries but no fractures or open wounds. The long-term needs will depend on the effect of the injury on soft tissue and internal organs and on the complication or comorbidity.

POTENTIAL HOME CARE PROBLEM

Alteration in role-relationship and potential for social isolation.

PLAN

Assess psychological effect of trauma on the ability of the older patient to continue to live in present situation.

REFERRAL INFORMATION

Referral to social services or elderly service agency for community follow-up should be done.

DRG 445

MDC 21   **RW$ 0.7530**   **Medical**   **Outlier Cutoff 25**   **Mean LOS 5.2**

Multiple Trauma – Age 18–69 w/o CC

DIAGNOSIS WITH POTENTIAL HOME CARE NEEDS

Multiple trauma

DETAILS TO CONSIDER

Patients listed in this group have multiple injuries but no fractures or open wounds. The long-term needs will depend on the effect of the injury on soft tissue and internal organs.

See **DRG 444.**

DRG 446

MDC 21   **RW$ 0.4846**   **Medical**   **Outlier Cutoff 10**   **Mean LOS 2.4**

Multiple Trauma – Age 0–17

DIAGNOSIS WITH POTENTIAL HOME CARE NEEDS

Multiple trauma

DETAILS TO CONSIDER

The reader is referred to pediatric references for additional information.

Allergic Reactions – Age > = 18

DIAGNOSES WITH POTENTIAL HOME CARE NEEDS

Anaphylactic shock
Angioneurotic edema
Allergy
Serum reaction

DETAILS TO CONSIDER

Very few patients are admitted to an acute care hospital in this group. Most of these diagnoses are treated in emergency rooms, urgent care centers or doctors' offices.

POTENTIAL HOME CARE PROBLEM

Health management deficit secondary to potential for subsequent reaction.

PLAN

Encourage patient with this severe allergic reaction to wear a Medic-Alert bracelet and notify primary physician of the reaction. Instruct patient in classification of substance or drug that caused the reaction to help avoid possibility of cross-allergy problems.

Allergic Reactions – Age 0–17

DIAGNOSIS WITH POTENTIAL HOME CARE NEEDS

Allergic reactions

See **DRG 447** and refer to pediatric references for additional information.

DRG 449

MDC 21	RW$ 0.7331	Medical	Outlier Cutoff 26	Mean LOS 5.6

Toxic Effects of Drugs – Age > = 70 and/or CC

DIAGNOSIS WITH POTENTIAL HOME CARE NEEDS

Toxic effects of drugs
Poisoning — any agent

DETAILS TO CONSIDER

The long-term needs of patients in this group will depend not only on monitoring drug intake but also on the complication and comorbidity. Drugs must be given to the elderly with great caution and with close follow-up. The elderly respond to medications and combinations of medications differently than do other age groups.

POTENTIAL HOME CARE PROBLEMS

PLAN

1. Health management deficit secondary to:

1a. need for multiple medications.

Evaluate all medications taken by the patient including over-the-counter drugs. Review total medication needs with the physician and pharmacist. Give the patient instructions in writing on medication plan.

1b. long-term effect of drug toxicity.

Assess impact of specific drug action on susceptible systems such as the liver or skin and instruct patient in follow-up care needed.

REFERRAL INFORMATION

A referral for a home care nurse is mandatory. Give detailed information on drug reaction and prescribed medications to be taken. Contact the patient's pharmacist who fills home use prescriptions and ask for a "unit-dose" type of dispenser. There are many available.

DRG 450

MDC 21	RW$ 0.5957	Medical	Outlier Cutoff 23	Mean LOS 3.9

Toxic Effects of Drugs – Age 18–69 w/o CC

DIAGNOSIS WITH POTENTIAL HOME CARE NEEDS

Toxic effects of drugs
Poisoning — any agent.

See **DRG 449.**

MDC 21	RW$ 0.2912	Medical	Outlier Cutoff 8	Mean LOS 2.1

Toxic Effects of Drugs – Age 0–17

DIAGNOSIS WITH POTENTIAL HOME CARE NEEDS

Toxic effects of drugs
Poisoning — any agent

DETAILS TO CONSIDER

The reader is referred to pediatric references for additional information.

MDC 21	RW$ 0.8492	Medical	Outlier Cutoff 26	Mean LOS 5.5

Complications of Treatment – Age > = 70 and/or CC

DIAGNOSES WITH POTENTIAL HOME CARE NEEDS

Malfunctioning device or graft
Postoperative wound disruption

DETAILS TO CONSIDER

The long-term needs will depend upon the type of device or upon the status of the postoperative wound. This is a medical admission; therefore there will not be a surgical intervention.

POTENTIAL HOME CARE PROBLEM

Health management deficit secondary to complication.

PLAN

Verify follow-up medical care. If patient was receiving home services prior to admission, reevaluate need. Communicate pertinent information to home health agency.

MDC 21	RW$ 0.9020	Medical	Outlier Cutoff 25	Mean LOS 5.1

Complications of Treatment – Age < 70 w/o CC

See **DRG 452**.

DRG 454

MDC 21	RW$ 0.8224	Medical	Outlier Cutoff 25	Mean LOS 5.3

Other Injuries, Poisonings and Toxic Effect Diagnoses
Age > = 70 and/or CC

DIAGNOSES WITH POTENTIAL HOME CARE NEEDS

Frostbite
Hypothermia
Hyperthermia
Asphyxiation
Maltreatment syndrome

DETAILS TO CONSIDER

Many of the diagnoses in this group result from exposure to the elements or from intentional abuse. The needs of the patient will depend on the long-term effect of the exposure, the amount of injury and the complication or comorbidity.

REFERRAL INFORMATION

Social services intervention is indicated for any patient with a diagnosis in this group, especially the elderly person.

DRG 455

MDC 21	RW$ 0.6185	Medical	Outlier Cutoff 22	Mean LOS 3.5

Other Injuries, Poisonings and Toxic Effect Diagnoses
Age < 70 w/o CC

See **DRG 454**.

22 MDC 22
BURNS: NOS*

***NOS = not otherwise specified as
Surgical or Medical (5 DRGs)**

Transferred to Another Acute Care Facility

Extensive Burns

Nonextensive with Skin Grafts

Nonextensive with Wound Debridement

There are 5 DRGs in **MDC 22.** Two of the DRGs are not classified as either **medical** or **surgical,** although burns of the body are most often treated by a surgeon. These 2 DRGs are not otherwise specified as **surgical** because there is no surgical procedure involved. The LOS ranges from 9.0– 18.3 and the relative weight ($) ranges from 1.4225 to 6.8631, **DRG 457,** giving it the distinction of being the highest weight of any DRG. Treating burns during the acute phase is very expensive because of the intensity of care and the multiple disciplines involved.

MASTER HOME CARE PLANNING GUIDE
FOR BURNS

Pattern	Assessment Factors	Plan
1. Alteration in skin integrity	Degree and depth of burn will affect the patient's skin healing and scar formation. In a young child extensive scarring and follow-up will be ongoing. Patient may also go home still requiring burn wound care.	Assess patient's and family's ability to do care of wound(s). Be sure specific wound care instructions are followed, especially if using topical agents.
2. Potential for wound infection	Assess condition of wound and bindings. Infection can convert a 2nd degree wound to 3rd degree. Carefully document appearance of burn wound on the discharge note.	Communicate appearance of wound to referral agency so that changes may be noted early. Teach patient and family aseptic technique.
3. Potential for alteration in self-image	Assess patient's coping mechanism and ability of patient and family to deal with the devastation of the burn wound and resultant scars.	Refer patient for psychiatric or psychological counseling.
4. Potential for drug abuse	Burn wounds, burn dressings and skin graft are usually associated with pain and thus pain control medications.	Assess patient's pain control regime and evaluate patient for potential addictive behavior.
5. Alteration in role-relationship	Patient is usually isolated for burn wound care and this can be psychologically damaging. Patient's burns may result in loss of job or family role change.	Assess patient's and family's ability to adapt change in lifestyle if necessary.
6. Alteration in nutritional needs	Burn patients need increased calories for healing. If child is burned, nutritional needs for growth and development must also be met.	Refer to dietician for instructions.
7. Potential joint contractures secondary to burn wounds	Assess joint involvement early. Assess patient's ability to carry out activities of daily living.	Early referral to occupational and physical therapy for splinting and mobilization of joints.

| MDC 22 | RW$ 2.0902 | Outlier Cutoff 32 | Mean LOS 11.6 |

Burns, Transferred to Another Acute Care Facility

DETAILS TO CONSIDER

The LOS in this DRG takes into account the time needed to stabilize an extensively burned patient. Following stabilization the patient will be transferred to another acute hospital, usually specializing in burn rehabilitation.

POTENTIAL HOME CARE PROBLEM

Potential for incomplete data transfer to referral hospital.

PLAN

Prepare adequate information to be sent with patient being transferred. Include along with present status, history of the injury, other injuries sustained, course of hospitalization, allergies, family status. Ideally a complete patient problem list including; medical, nursing, social therapy and dietary input.

REFERRAL INFORMATION

Depending on the location of the hospital to which the patient is transferred, the family will need help and counseling in meeting the needs of the family. Rehabilitation hospital **Length of Stay** and **DRG** payment should be investigated at the time of discharge so the patient, family and caregivers will be aware of payment mechanism.

DRG 457

MDC 22	RW$ 6.8631	Outlier Cutoff 33	Mean LOS 12.6

Extensive Burns (not otherwise specified)

DETAILS TO CONSIDER

Extensive burns take into consideration the size of the burn, the degree and part of the body involved. For example, a 20% 3rd Degree burn is considered extensive. The variations of degree and percentage in this DRG are understandably many. The primary goal of hospital treatment is fluid stability and healing of full-thickness burns. This DRG does not include skin grafting.

POTENTIAL HOME CARE PROBLEM

Wound care due to incomplete healing of 1st and 2nd degree wounds.

PLAN

Teach patient and family wound care. Location of wound will have impact on referral needs. If patient manages wound, allow patient to do dressings as method of teaching.

REFERRAL INFORMATION

Again, depending on part of body involved, referral needs will vary. Minimal needs are for a home care nurse to monitor healing process and follow-up care. Referral needs may include occupational therapy, physical therapy and medical social service. If necessary, durable medical equipment such as hospital bed, walker or cane may be needed. Splints and braces may be needed if joints are affected. Medical/surgical supplies need to be ordered — such as dressing and topicals.

DRG 458

MDC 22	RW$ 2.8572	Surgical	Outlier Cutoff 38	Mean LOS 18.3

Nonextensive Burns with Skin Grafts

DETAILS TO CONSIDER

Burns in this DRG may not cover large body surfaces but are deep and require grafting to cover.

See **Master Care Plan** and **DRG 457**.

POTENTIAL HOME CARE PROBLEMS

1. Donor site wound care.

2. Alteration in body image.

PLAN

Type of care depends on physician's choice. Some donor sites are left open to heal or can be covered with fine mesh gauze.

Discuss with patient future plans for cosmetic surgery if grafted area is visible. Immediate appearance of graft may be upsetting. Discuss healing process of wound.

REFERRAL INFORMATION

See **DRG 457**.

| MDC 22 | RW$ 2.7568 | Surgical | Outlier Cutoff 33 | Mean LOS 12.7 |

Nonextensive Burns with Wound Debridement and Other Operating Room Procedures

DETAILS TO CONSIDER

Wound debridement can be done at the bedside, so the patient may not need to go to the operating room. Eschar, the scab-like tissue, has no nerve supply; therefore debridement should not be very painful. Adequate documentation of wound debridement in the progress notes is essential. No operative note will be available if procedure is done at the bedside and DRG grouping depends on debridement information.

REFERRAL INFORMATION

See **DRG 457.**

| MDC 22 | RW$ 1.4225 | Medical | Outlier Cutoff 29 | Mean LOS 9.0 |

Nonextensive Burns w/o OR Procedure

DETAILS TO CONSIDER

Burns of head and neck with resultant respiratory involvement may be considered nonextensive but require relatively long hospitalization for treatment. Burns of the perineum and genital area also do not cover a large percentage of body surface but require intense care.

POTENTIAL HOME CARE PROBLEMS

PLAN

1. Alteration in respiratory status.

Evaluate patient's respiratory status and need for follow-up care. Smoke inhalation can lead to pneumonitis and pneumonia. If there was airway obstruction at the time of injury or patient required endotracheal intubation, monitoring for possible long-term effects is indicated.

2. Potential alteration in elimination secondary to perineal burns.

Instruct patient in good toileting habits. Wounds in the perineum frequently become infected because of fecal contamination. A Foley catheter may have been used for fluid monitoring due to swelling of the meatus.

REFERRAL INFORMATION

Medical follow-up is essential if patient had respiratory or perineal burns. Referral needs for a home care nurse will depend on the patient's progress, but usually are not necessary.

23

MDC 23
FACTORS INFLUENCING HEALTH STATUS AND OTHER CONTACTS WITH HEALTH SERVICES

SURGICAL GROUPINGS (1 DRG)

Operating Room Procedures

MEDICAL GROUPINGS (6 DRGs)

Rehabilitation

Signs and Symptoms

Aftercare

Aftercare with History of Malignancy as Secondary Diagnosis

Other Factors Influencing Health Care

The diagnoses in this MDC are grouped together in a miscellaneous manner; therefore there can be no Master Care Plan because of the variety of problems.

See each DRG for information.

DRG 461   DRG 461

MDC 23	RW$ 1.6507	Surgical	Outlier Cutoff 28	Mean LOS 8.0

Operating Room Procedures with Diagnoses of Other Contacts with Health Services

DETAILS TO CONSIDER

For planning purposes refer to the DRG that includes the operative procedure.

DRG 462   DRG 462

MDC 23	RW$ 1.8268	Medical	Outlier Cutoff 34	Mean LOS 13.5

Rehabilitation

DIAGNOSES WITH POTENTIAL HOME CARE NEEDS

Prosthetic fitting
Physical therapy
Occupational therapy
Speech therapy

DETAILS TO CONSIDER

The consideration for home care needs will not only depend on the diagnosis of "rehabilitation" but on the underlying diagnosis and on the general health status of the patient. Conditions such as cardiovascular, cerebrovascular and neurological disease will also affect the long-term needs of the patient. In this DRG the Care Plan will list areas to be addressed in making the decision for follow-up care.

POTENTIAL HOME CARE PROBLEMS

1. Health management deficit.

PLAN

Can the patient and caregiver manage the care of the patient? Is there a potential for injury, such as falling, for both the patient and caregiver? Is there potential for noncompliance with health care plan because of noncaring attitude, finances or unavailability of services? Is there a potential for complications from inappropriate use of medications or from inability to carry out medical plan?

2. Alteration in nutrition.

Will patient be able to receive prescribed diet and fluids on a regular basis? Will the patient's skin integrity be compromised from inadequate nutrition? Do the patient and family understand the prescribed diet? Does the patient need assistive devices? Can he/she swallow without potential for aspiration?

3. Alteration in elimination.

Is the patient able to manage bowel and bladder function at a safe level? Does the caregiver understand the bowel and bladder routine? Are the toileting facilities convenient?

4. Interruption in activity/exercise pattern secondary to impaired mobility.

Can the patient ambulate or transfer safely either alone or with minimal assistance? Does the patient need a mechanical device such as a Hoyer lift for transfer? Is there a prosthetic or orthotic device involved? Do the patient and caregiver know how to use and care for the device? Do the patient and caregiver have instructions in activities and exercises to prevent contractures?

5. Alteration in cognitive pattern.

Is a pain management plan in place and is the patient relatively pain-free? Can the patient communicate? Is it safe to leave the patient alone if he/she has a communication deficit? Can the patient think clearly and does he/she have an attention span that allows for completion of a task or decision making? Does the patient and family understand the diagnosis and prognosis?

6. Sleep pattern disturbance.

Is the patient's bed easy to get to, get into and out of, have a comfortable mattress and safety features? Does the patient need a hospital bed with a trapeze and side rails? Can the patient sleep with the usual sleeping partner? Will the caregiver get ample sleep and rest?

7. Anxiety related to self-preparation and alteration in body image.

How is the patient handling the change in body image; has he/she begun to resolve the personal identity changes related to the diagnosis? What will the long-term needs of the patient be in terms of acceptance of physical change in appearance and behavior changes?

8. Independence/dependence conflict.

What was the patient's level of functioning prior to hospitalization? Will there be a change in a parenting or spousal relationship because of dependency? Will the socialization needs of patient and family be able to be met? Does the verbal ability affect social relationships? Is the speech pattern and comprehension level different? Is there a potential for physical or verbal abuse, or neglect of the patient because of the severity of the handicap?

9. Alteration in sexuality and reproductive pattern.

What effect does the diagnosis have on the patient's ability to participate in sexual activity? Is there a potential for an unplanned pregnancy? Can the female patient manage personal hygiene needs during her menstrual cycle?

10. Potential for ineffective coping resulting in family stress.

Have the patient and family begun to deal with impact of illness on all phases of family living? Have they addressed changes in all functional patterns listed above? Do they know where to get counseling on a long-term basis?

REFERRAL INFORMATION

All of the diagnoses in this DRG will require follow-up care. In some cases the patient may be home-bound for a period of time and thus will be eligible for home care. Also in some cases the patient can and should receive services in an out-patient setting. Insurance for these services varies from policy to policy. A careful investigation into covered services is vital. Medicare has stringent eligibility criteria by which they review bills for rehabilitation services.

The hospital designation must meet specific criteria set by HCFA (Health Care Financing Administration) and the payment mechanism depends on this status. Not all rehabilitation hospitals nor rehabilitation units meet this cirteria; therefore the billing mechanism is the same for any other diagnosis. If you're not sure of your status, check with your Administrator, Business Office or Medical Records Department.

If your hospital is not designated as a rehabilitation hospital or if you do not have a distinct rehabilitation unit, then the patient may be eligible for transfer to a rehabilitation setting. Patient's needs when discharged from a rehabilitation admission must be clearly defined. If the patient is **NOT HOME BOUND** then arrangements for outpatient therapy must be made. It is important to note that Home Health Agencies providing services must attest in writing to the **HOME BOUND** status and document **WHY** the patient is home bound.

Patients with the following diagnoses qualify as needing hospital level rehabilitation: stroke; spinal cord injury; congenital deformity; amputation; major multiple trauma; fracture of the femur (also called hip fracture); brain injury; polyarthritis including rheumatoid arthritis. Additional services include social services.

The length of stay is a relatively short 13.5 for patients who need rehabilitation; therefore plans for admission to a rehabilitation hospital or distinct unit should be made early. The decision to send the patient home for rehabilitation should include consideration for the intensity of service. If the patient meets the homebound criteria and needs therapy no more than once a day and does not need close medical supervision he/she may be a candidate. Patient safety must be a primary concern. Multidisciplinary conferences should be held to make long-term decisions about the patient. The family or primary caregiver must be involved in the decision making process.

MDC 23 **RW$ 0.7702** **Medical** **Outlier Cutoff 26** **Mean LOS 6.3**

Signs and Symptoms with CC

General symptoms (e.g. edema, cyanosis, etc.)

DETAILS TO CONSIDER

The long-term needs will depend on the etiology of the symptoms. Very few patients are admitted in this DRG; most are admitted with a medical diagnosis with these symptoms listed as secondary problems. However, the patient may present themselves to an emergency room with these symptoms never having been diagnosed.

POTENTIAL HOME CARE PROBLEM

Health management deficit secondary to life-threatening symptom.

PLAN

Arrangements made for medical follow-up for patients admitted through the emergency room or who do not have a primary physician.

MDC 23 **RW$ 0.7322** **Medical** **Outlier Cutoff 26** **Mean LOS 6.0**

Signs and Symptoms w/o CC

Same as **DRG 463**.

DRG 465

MDC 23	RW$ 0.2071	Medical	Outlier Cutoff 4	Mean LOS 1.5

Aftercare with History of Malignancy as Secondary Diagnosis

DETAILS TO CONSIDER

Patients in this DRG are most often admitted to the hospital for a diagnostic test or therapy that cannot be done on an outpatient basis.

POTENTIAL HOME CARE PROBLEM

Health management deficit.

PLAN

Determine the changes in the patient's needs related to the diagnostic findings or to the reaction to the therapy. Refer to DRGs discussing the patient's underlying diagnosis.

REFERRAL INFORMATION

If the patient is already receiving home services, be sure to communicate any new information to the nurse or therapist caring for the patient.

DRG 466

MDC 23	RW$ 0.6377	Medical	Outlier Cutoff 24	Mean LOS 3.7

Aftercare w/o History of Malignancy as Secondary Diagnosis

DETAILS TO CONSIDER

See DRG 465.

DRG 467

MDC 23	RW$ 0.9799	Medical	Outlier Cutoff 26	Mean LOS 6.1

Other Factors Influencing Health Status

DIAGNOSES WITH POTENTIAL HOME CARE NEEDS

Contact with infectious agent
History of major illness
Screening for major illness

DETAILS TO CONSIDER

This DRG is one that is frequently assigned to patients admitted with a medical condition which cannot be grouped into another more specific DRG. The long-term needs will depend on the patient's specific major illness.

See related DRGs.

24 UNGROUPABLE DRG'S

Not all patients can be assigned to a DRG. If a patient's medical records abstract contains invalid information or if the clinical information on the abstract contains certain types of inconsistencies, then the patient may not be assigned to one of the 467 DRGs. Three additional patient classes have been defined to identify the situations in which a patient will not be assigned to one of the DRGs.

Patients who cannot be assigned to a DRG are given a patient class number of 468, 469 or 470.

DRG 468

RW$ 2.1037   **Not Specified**   **Outlier Cutoff 31**   **Mean LOS 11.2**

Unrelated Operating Room Procedure

DETAILS TO CONSIDER

Patients are assigned to **DRG 468** when all the operating room procedures performed are unrelated to the patient's principal diagnosis. This assignment can be the result of coding error, but may also be the result of an accurate coding. In these cases, patients who are admitted for a particular diagnosis develop a complication unrelated to the principal diagnosis and thus have an operating room procedure performed for this complication.

DRG 469

RW$ Not Applicable   **Not Specified**   **Outlier Cutoff 0**   **Mean LOS 0**

Principal Diagnosis Invalid as Discharge Diagnosis

DETAILS TO CONSIDER

Patients are assigned to **DRG 469** when a principal diagnosis is coded which is not precise enough to allow the patient to be assigned to a DRG.

DRG 470

RW$ Not Applicable   **Not Specified**   **Outlier Cutoff 0**   **Mean LOS 0**

Ungroupable

DETAILS TO CONSIDER

Patients are assigned to **DRG 470** if certain types of medical record problems which may affect DRG assignment are present. Patients with an invalid or nonexistent code as a principal diagnosis will be assigned to **DRG 470**.

BIBLIOGRAPHY

Averill, ICDM-9-CM Diagnosis Related Group, Health Systems International New Haven. 1984.

Birmingham. J. Medical Terminology: A Self Learning Module. McGraw-Hill Book Co., New York. 1981.

Benenson, A. S. Control of Communicable Disease in Man. American Public Health Association, Washington, D.C. 1980.

Bradley, E. L. Complications of Pancreatitis. W. B. Saunders Co., Philadelphia. 1982.

Brain, M., and P. McCulloch. Current Therapy in Hematology-Oncology 1983–1984. C. V. Mosby Co., St. Louis. 1983.

Brooks, F. Diseases of the Exocrine Pancreas. W. B. Saunders Co., Philadelphia. 1980.

Campbell, J. W., and M. Frisse, editors. Manual of Medical Therapeutics. Little, Brown & Co., Boston. 1983. Twenty-fourth edition.

Cassileth, B. R. The Cancer Patient: Social and Medical Aspects of Care. Lea & Febiger, Philadelphia. 1979.

Gordon, M. Nursing Diagnosis: Process and Application. McGraw-Hill Book Co., New YorK. 1982.

Havener, W. H. Synopsis of Ophthalmology. C. V. Mosby Co., St. Louis. 1979. Fifth edition.

Health Care Financing Administration (HCFA), Department of Health and Human Services Medicare Program: Prospective Payments for Medicare Inpatient Hospital Services. Federal Register (September 1, 1983). 39752–39890.

Health Care Financing Administration (HCFA), Department of Health and Human Services: Final rule. Federal Register (January 3, 1984). 234–334.

Hills, S. W., and J. J. Birmingham: Burn Care. John Wiley & Sons, Inc., New York. 1981.

Howe, J., et al: The Handbook of Nursing. John Wiley & Sons, Inc., New York. 1984.

Kaufman, J. J. Current Urologic Therapy. W. B. Saunders Co., Philadelphia. 1980.

Orr, M. E. Acute Pancreatic and Hepatic Dysfunction. John Wiley & Sons, Inc., New York, 1981.

Rubin, P. Clinical Oncology for Medical Students and Physicians. American Cancer Society, New York. 1983. Sixth edition.

Smith, D. R. General Urology. Lange Medical Publications, Los Altos, Calif. 1981. Tenth edition.

Snyder, M., editor. A Guide to Neurological and Neurosurgical Nursing. John Wiley & Sons Inc., New York. 1983.

Steinberg, F. U. Care of the Geriatric Patient. C. V. Mosby Co., St. Louis. 1983.

Taylor, J. W., and S. Ballenger. Neurological Dysfunctions and Nursing Intervention. McGraw-Hill Book Co., New York. 1980.

Waterbury, L. Hematology for the House Officer. Williams & Wilkins Co., Baltimore. 1981.